Economics and Nature

Essays in Balance, Complementarity and Harmony

Economics and Nature

Essays in Balance, Complementarity and Harmony

Navin Doshi

with a Foreword by
Ravi Batra

Nalanda International
Los Angeles (USA)

PRINTWORLD
Publishers of Indian Traditions

Cataloging in Publication Data — DK
[Courtesy: D.K. Agencies (P) Ltd. <docinfo@dkagencies.com>]

Doshi, Navin.
Economics and nature : essays in balance, complementarity and harmony / Navin Doshi ; with a foreword by Ravi Batra.
p. cm.
Includes bibliographical references (p.) and index.
ISBN 13: 9788124606223

1. Economic history. 2. Financial crises. 3. International economic relations. I. Title.

DDC 338.927 23

ISBN 13: 978-81-246-0622-3 (Hb) ISBN 10: 81-246-0622-6
ISBN 13: 978-81-246-0624-7 (Pb) ISBN 10: 81-246-0624-2
First published in India in 2012

Published by:
Nalanda Interantional
"Nalanda", 64818, Spring Park Avenue
Los Angeles, CA - 90056 (USA)
Phones: (310)-430-8057; *Fax*: (213)-341 0156
Web: www.nalandainternational.com

and

D.K. Printworld (P) Ltd.
Regd. Office : *'Vedaśrī'*, F-395, Sudarshan Park
(Metro Station: Ramesh Nagar)
New Delhi - 110 015
Phones : (011) 2545 3975; 2546 6019; *Fax* : (011) 2546 5926
E-mail : indology@dkprintworld.com
Web : www.dkprintworld.com

Printed by: D.K. Printworld (P) Ltd., New Delhi

Foreword

Ever since 2007, when home prices began to sink in the United States, the American economy has varied from stagnation to a deep recession. According to official claims the slump ended in 2009, but large-scale unemployment has persisted with little hope in sight. Naturally, people are wondering what is wrong with the state of the US and global economy, where even trillion dollar budget deficits and corporate bailouts have been unable to fix the problem. Several economists have offered a variety of cures, but unfortunately their remedies are old-fashioned and are unable to meet the new challenges.

It is in this troublesome background that Navin Doshi has written a book, which, in my view, offers a better explanation and cures than most competing works. Each and every chapter of *Economics and Nature* emits freshness lacking in similar books written in recent years. Navin is no economist, which seems to be a blessing in itself, because most of today's established economists start out with an agenda and then look for theories to rationalise their preconceived notions. That is why the globe finds itself ridden with intractable problems. Those theories are now obsolete and have to be discarded. Navin, by contrast, has a business and engineering background, and he offers an approach based on common sense and human nature.

There are a lot of imbalances in the world today, but modern economists and governments try to eliminate one imbalance by creating another. For instance, the American consumer is drowning in debt, but to mitigate the effects of this excess the US government is creating another pile of debt. As if one mountain of debt is not bad enough. Similarly, the top bankers and CEOs of major corporations earn billions every year, yet the government and the Federal Reserve have bailed them out again and again, putting billions more into their pockets. Thus, one imbalance is being neutralised by another, and this cannot be the right cure. It may postpone the sickness for a while, but the malady will return with force.

Navin puts his faith in the laws of nature, which ensures that imbalances don't persist for long. Otherwise, there are violent consequences in the form of tornadoes, hurricanes and earthquakes. Economies also exist in nature and have to follow its immutable laws. For economic wisdom Navin looks to the ancient past, when the debt piles that afflict nations today were not possible, so that people had to solve their financial problems by correcting the fundamentals and not just apply band-aids to festering wounds. He discovers that the first great economist was an Indian luminary named Kautilya, who, as the prime minister of a great empire, had to revive an economy ravaged by wars and droughts. Kautilya turns out to be a modern version of John Maynard Keynes, whose ideas underlie much of the fixes that the governments are using currently around the world. But Navin finds that Keynesian economics has been totally misinterpreted, because Keynes never condoned a relentless rise in government debt and printing of money.

Navin is not an ideologue. That is why, unlike many others, he finds no contradiction between Keynes and Milton Friedman. While Keynes offered a cure for an economy in a recession or depression, Friedman suggested remedies to fight inflation. Combining the wisdom of the two offers a balanced economic policy that Navin advocates.

Navin is a concerned individual. He is concerned that vast global imbalances of today will rupture again and land the world in another recession. He is concerned that millions of investors could lose their savings yet again, and millions more could join the army of the unemployed. He is worried that we are compounding the problems created by the most recent Great Recession, and wasting precious time in not offering genuine economic reforms.

In short, *Economics and Nature* by Navin Doshi is a serious work written by a man of integrity and business acumen, who is concerned about the well-being of our society. He wants to rejuvenate the economy by combining the wisdom of the past with practical and logical policies offered by some wise economists today.

Dallas, Texas **Ravi Batra**
15 September 2011

Preface

This book in essence is a by-product of my first book, *Transcendence . . . Saving Us From Ourselves*. We humans have come a long way to learning and understanding nature within and without. Before we go into the subject of economy, let me describe what I have understood based upon the works of two theoretical physicists Amit Goswami and Ulrich Mohrhoff, working independently and geographically poles apart. Their work implies an affirmation of the Vedantic tradition that there is an ultimate self-conscious reality. This reality is the world and the cosmos we live in, it is also the consciousness that contains and penetrates the cosmos in its totality. This ultimate reality is, subjectively speaking, an infinite bliss, and objectively speaking, an infinite in any quality and value we can imagine that expresses and experiences itself. This follows the top-down framework of the Vedantic kind with quality, value and consciousness rooted in the very heart of Reality, as opposed to the bottom-up framework of the materialist kind with no idealism or sentience attached to it. Please note that the universe exists by itself in the material sense, and it exists for itself is in the sense of consciousness. I also interpret, based upon their findings, that there is non-local, meaning beyond the realm of perceivable space and time, quantum connection between individual subjective consciousness and the all-pervading objective super-consciousness. It has also been accepted that the nature within and without is fractal, meaning it is layered like an onion, and in which each part contains the whole. The implication here is that, not only our mind, but Consciousness itself is layered and has discrete poises rising towards greater consciousness and wholeness. Sri Aurobindo had pioneered this subject and claimed that humanity is on the evolutionary path of transcendence towards the Ultimate Reality.

We need an economic arrangement that will not only facilitate but also help accelerate the process of transcendence as described above. It is easier for me to explain a good economic system by reciting my own story. I was born in India in the year 1936, when the freedom movement under the leadership of great men like Mahatma Gandhi was in full swing. Many teachers in my high school were followers of Gandhi and believed in Gandhi's idealism of simple living. I had, along with my family, an opportunity to spend an afternoon with Mahatma Gandhi, walking and participating in evening prayers; I was about 10 years old. In subsequent years, based upon my own interest and counselling, I received a degree in mechanical engineering in India (1958) and came to America for higher education. After finishing the Masters degree, I worked as an aerospace engineer for about two and half decades. Later on, I initiated my own business in textiles, real estate and financial investment. Over time, I achieved my goal of becoming financially independent in America.

Though I am not an economist by training, I taught myself about economics based on experience and self-learning. So, what is an ideal economic arrangement? Call it Capitalism or a Free Enterprise system, it is the most natural economic arrangement that I know, where anyone has an opportunity to succeed. But, it needs the promotion of an ethical consciousness to work. Corruption and too much government intrusion become its Achilles' heel. I had little chance to succeed in India, at least in the 1970s, due to too much government interference and corruption. India's economic growth started to accelerate only after government intrusion began receding in the early 1990s. The economic system in America has been admired because almost anyone with some creative idea, has a good chance to succeed even today. I remember how someone succeeded selling pet rocks. On each rock was painted a unique facial expression, and attached to each rock was a card with a few good words.

As described by the journalist Thomas Friedman in his book, *That Used to be Us . . .*, the five pillars that made America the most powerful country, were:

(1) Open-ended education system.

(2) Immigration policy that brought in the best minds and most talented people from other countries.

(3) Building the best infrastructure.

(4) Government working in partnership with the private sector, and providing incentives for capital formation, and risk-taking with rules to prevent recklessness.

(5) Government-funded research.

Those were the good days with good work ethics, and most Americans had high respect for the government. I had come across a few Americans who believed that not paying taxes was not only unethical but also sinful. The socio-political events like the Watergate scandal, disconnect from the gold standard, Vietnam and Yom Kippur wars, affected the economy adversely. The misery index composed of the interest rate, unemployment rate, and the CPI index, went up to the moon. Both husband and wife started to work to keep up with the "Joneses", but it also affected raising children adversely. Today the economy, not only in America but also in many European countries, is in the worst condition due to several reasons including enormous government debt and spending deficit, unfavourable demographics and unrestrained greed. "Too Big to Fail" banks with little government supervision are also responsible for creating economic polarisation.

I have described in this book the ways of bringing balance between two economic opposites, bringing harmony between the two. Often, opposites need to work together complementing each other, instead of destroying the nemesis. For a solution to inequalities, a clear perception of the problems is first necessary. It seems every pair, liberals and conservatives, labour and management, paper currencies and inflation hedges, and many more . . . all seem to be out of balance. Then, there are problems of corruption at the highest levels in India and Gaponomics, implying widening gap between the rich and the poor in Western countries. What we need is life-education, not merely professional education without morality, which has led us to the exploitative world of today, but the education of the heart. We need to put more emphasis on such education at every level. Education that unifies humanity, but maintains individual autonomy, that stimulates the highest level of creativity, should become our universal currency of the mind, with more positive results. The Holy Grail in every human endeavour is unification, as for example, unification of all forces in physics. I believe a good natural economic system will help fulfil all somatic and philosophic desires of men, leaving only one desire, and that desire would be the desire of becoming selfless. A "superconducting" economy, where resistance to the flow of money, the misery index, and unemployment index is close to zero and the somatic needs of all are totally satisfied. Humanity needs to accelerate the evolutionary processes within to make us more humanitarian, more ethical, more responsible, more detached, more compassionate, and more loving. The political and economic systems have to be such that they are natural, providing a path of our choice for the final destination.

This book is divided in two parts; the first part is about the history and the theory of economic systems going back 2000 years ago, and the second part contains essays about what has happened in matters of economics in last several years in America. One can get the flavour of the book by reviewing the aphorisms given in Appendix A. Market clichés associated with the laws of nature are given in Appendix B.

I wish to thank Professor Ravi Batra for his valuable insights and advice and for writing the Foreword. I also wish to thank my wife Pratima Doshi and my colleague Debashish Banerji for their encouragement and support.

Navin Doshi

Contents

Opinions !

Bravo! Overall, this provides an excellent layperson's overview of economic history for the past century. Every reader can relate to the primary theme: let's take a good long look at the story of money and understand how our actions must be guided by prudence and common sense. As Navin Doshi insightfully writes: "You cannot defy the laws of addition and subtraction!"

Christopher Key Chapple, Ph.D.
Professor of Indic and Comparative Theology
Loyola Marymount University
Editor, *Worldviews: Global Religions, Culture, and Ecology*
bestselling author of books on Yoga Philosophy

When a highly trained aeronautical engineer has his feet firmly grounded in economic and psychological realities, he can look far and deep into life. Navin Doshi is such a person for whom Nature, seen through the twin eyes of Western science and Indian philosophy, from outside in and inside out, offers pointers to our economic well-being. *Economics and Nature* is his book that interrogates the harsh economic actualities of the present and searches for pathways to harmony in personal, familial and social life.

Sitanshu Yashaschandra, Ph.D.
Former Vice-chancellor, Saurashtra University
UGC Emeritus Professor, and National Lecturer
Chief Editor, *Encyclopaedia of Indian Literature*

Navin Doshi's astute grasp of nature, history and psychology allows him to penetrate the American economic crisis of our times and provide solutions for individual and social survival and well being. In today's global interdependent world, this is a book which carries understanding and practical wisdom for everyone.

Debashish Banerji, Ph.D.
Professor of Indian Studies, and
Dean of Academic Affairs
University of Philosophical Research, Los Angeles

Part I
Economics and Nature

1

Good Economy: An Introduction

It is a well-known dictum of history that reform movements and great new systems are born in the cradle of major crises. People remain complacent and busy with routine life until they are faced with a challenging milieu. Sometimes, even challenges don't budge them. Then upheavals occur to shake them out of their torpor. It appears to me that humanity is passing through another crisis today, and if we don't wake up in time it could turn into an ugly upheaval and great hardship for all.

Let us take a close but objective look at the global economy. There are a lot of success stories to talk about. Following Second World War, a great mass of people lived in poverty while the United States, Canada and Australia emerged not only as victors from the War but also with a much larger industrial base than ever before. However, the rest of the world faced devastation, even disease and hunger. The War had destroyed the once flourishing economies of Europe and Japan. The Middle East, India and other parts of Asia were beset with famines, whereas China was mired in a nation's ultimate calamity — a long and bloody civil war.

Just prior to Second World War, the world shivered in the chills of the Great Depression. A great pall of gloom and doom hung over most nations, except Germany and Japan, the very nations that had been arming themselves to start hostilities. The War devastated much of the globe, but the trio of the United States, Canada and Australia saw their depression end and more than regained their economic heights.

A lot has happened since then, especially in the realm of politics and technology. We have actually moved on to a new millennium, which itself is a momentous occurrence, at least chronologically. India is now free, in fact, became so in 1947, soon after the War; China is a superpower, economically and militarily. Gone are the days when the nation could be bullied by Western powers and neighbouring Japan. Ask an octogenarian Chinese, and he/she would simply marvel at the transformation of his or her nation. In fact, my usage of he/she to represent a person itself is an astounding change that separates us from a practice that lingered for thousands of years. Women have come a long way in much of the planet, and at least in the West, they frown upon the word "man" representing both a man and a woman. Yet the practice prevails in much of the world, especially among scholars.

The Soviet Union is no more; nor is the Shah of Iran, the supreme head of that nation. The two Germanys have become one, with East Germany integrated into one German nation. South Africa is no longer ruled by a white minority practising apartheid. Above all, the globe is knit into a single fabric through a technological revolution that rivals some of the greatest innovations ever in history. Computers, the Internet, the cell phone, the fax, among countless others have transformed the world into a global village. Few countries can keep secrets for long. News travels fast, as do people and goods across nations.

Surging international trade has rearranged economies. China has emerged as the export locomotive of the world, and its trade surplus obtained from low cost labour has killed the power of labour unions in the United States and weakened them elsewhere. No longer is America the sole economic powerhouse; in fact, it resembles a banana republic in many respects.

Man has already visited the moon, and space probes regularly land on the Mars. Some even suggest that interplanetary travel is not far off. Astronauts periodically live for months in deep space, transmit fascinating pictures of earth from afar. On the seamy side, glaciers are beginning to meltdown, and many fear that low lying areas will be inundated in our lifetime.

Myriad changes have occurred from the pre-Second World War days, but one thing has not changed — the human tendency to create its own imbalances and problems. For some reason, we are not content with a smooth functioning of the economy and society for long. Human history is a thrilling novel of ups and downs. Good days seem to sow seeds of a crisis, which wakes us up and forces us to look for reforms. Then recovery occurs, good days return, but within a few years reforms give rise to loopholes that are exploited by some, and another crisis inevitably returns. This way we move along a roller-coaster of history.

Let us examine the economic history of the twentieth century. The American economy was fairly prosperous from 1900 to 1920, with a minor downturn in 1907. Europe, Japan and Asia also faced relatively few problems. The world economy and share markets moved more or less smoothly during this period. Then came the Roaring Twenties, when great imbalances occurred not just in the United States, but also in other parts of the world. Share prices in North America, Europe and Australia zoomed and turned maniacal, consumer debt soared almost everywhere, foreign commerce displayed large deficits or surpluses, and real earnings lagged behind productivity growth in most nations. These were the germs of an impending crisis, which built up over a decade. Then came the 1930s, and the global economy collapsed. The imbalances of the preceding decade were not planetary, as some nations, such as India and China escaped them, but the collapse was worldwide.

Nations came to recognise the excesses of the 1920s, but it was too late. The Great Depression had already begun at the end of that decade. Unemployment soared, crime multiplied, hunger, homelessness and despair stalked the globe. None of this resulted from natural calamities; the depression was a man-made calamity. So the solutions too had to be man-made. Belatedly, a variety of reforms were instituted in Europe, Australia and North America to restore prosperity and then to avoid the return of the slump, but to no avail.

So deep was the downturn that in the United States the economy was simply overhauled. New institutions emerged while old ones were tightly regulated. Social security, unemployment compensation and minimum wage were legislated for the first time. Share markets and banks were brought under tight control. However, nothing worked for a while. The US economy stabilised after 1933, but remained mired in the Depression. Its joblessness was still above 18 per cent at the end of the decade. Eventually, the depression ended not because of economic reforms, but because of Second World War.

Who knows how long the Depression would have lasted if it were not for the start of war by Adolf Hitler? The point of the matter is that even a calamity such as the Great Depression did not move the nation to create an economy that would improve by itself. Indeed, many reforms were introduced, but they could not end the debacle. We need an economic system that is self-healing, a system that adjusts to its environment maintaining balance and harmony with nature, deviating not too far from the sweetest spot in a multidimensional space created by Nature. It inherently generates prosperity for all and can withstand a variety of pressures. In other words, we need to create an ideal economy.

An Ideal Economy

Why do we want to explore an ideal economy? It is because

first of all, modern economy runs on money, a vehicle of exchange, and money is the mother's milk of everything, not just of politics, as Jesse Unruh, the celebrated speaker of California's Assembly, once stated in 1960. All of God's creatures believe in one religion, the religion of survival. The human survival, at almost every level, depends upon money. The human body is the mother of the mind, a necessary instrument to think, philosophise, and to transcend to a higher state of being. It seems to me that an idealised economy could only come from an idealised mind. Prince Siddhartha was fortunate to be born in a royal family; there was no reason for him to be concerned about the needs of his somatic self. When he observed an old man with a decaying body, realising the impermanence of human existence, he went through gruelling penance for years to search and discover a permanent abode that he later called *nirvana*. Only then he transcended, passing through various states of mind, to the state of the Buddha. He then possessed an ideal mind that offered a way to create an ideal society, a middle way and away from extremes of pleasure and pain. Thus, an ideal economy should be able to offer resources to those who are interested in developing a higher state of mind.

The ideal economy imperative is as strong today as ever. Global imbalances towards the end of the first decade of the twenty-first century are worse than those at the end of the 1920s. At least in the past, nations did not have huge debts. Today there is hardly any country whose government is free from financial burdens. Governments now borrow during good and bad times. They borrow less when the economy is prosperous and more when it is slumping, but they always borrow.

The global environment was also less toxic in the past. Today the rivers, the seas, the lakes, the skies, and furthermore, land are all polluted. The 1920s suffered from great concentration of wealth. Things are no better today.

Then, as now, there was large-scale poverty on earth. Then, as now, trade imbalances were vast and growing. Above all, the gap between labour productivity and people's salaries is perhaps higher than ever. Wages are not that low, but productivity is the highest in history, so the chasm between earnings and efficiency is arguably worse today than in the past. Wherever there is smoke there is fire; so wherever there are imbalances, there is a potential crisis. And that is what motivates me to write this book, to discover an ideal economy that is immune from imbalances, and stays near the sweet spot between two extremes.

I hope I am considered sufficiently qualified to undertake this task, mostly because, I dare say, I am not an economist by qualification. I have been a lifelong student of science, economics, philosophy, psychology and life itself. I have a Masters degree in engineering, and am now a semi-retired businessman by profession. I have spent a lot of time reflecting on the problems plaguing our nation and the globe today. Some of the best economic ideas have come from non-economists, perhaps because they possess strong common sense that is free from inherited beliefs or the ideology of the time. The celebrated idea of free trade came from David Ricardo, an English businessman. By contrast, the best economic minds of the 1930s could not produce a system that by itself would move out of the Depression. As described above, it was the Second World War, not the established economists that ended the decade-long slump. It appears that common sense, together with reformist ideas available from non-partisan sources, trumps a high diploma any day when it comes to a good economy.

Throughout history, good economic ideas have either come from philosophers, businessmen, or maverick economists, who took refuge in common sense but were denounced by their peers. Take, for instance, John Maynard Keynes, who offered a theory that is commonly known as Keynesian economics. His ideas underlie much of economic policy practised by our government today, although like any good medicine they have been overused, even abused, much to the detriment of our economy.

When Fed chairman, Ben Bernanke, began cutting interest rates in 2007, he simply emulated Keynes to ward off a recession. When another Fed chairman, Paul Volcker, raised interest rates to fight inflation in the early 1980s, he followed Milton Friedman but also Keynes. Friedman is known as an inflation fighter, but it was Keynes, who first explained the process in which monetary restraint first raises the rate of interest, then crimps investment and consumer demand, and finally tames inflation. Keynes was against the gold standard, because he wanted a flexible monetary policy to fight recessions, but he constantly warned the world against excessive printing of money to avoid high inflation. When President Kennedy cut taxes, mostly for the middle class in the early 1960s, to combat unemployment, he translated Keynesian economics into practical government policy. So Keynes is the mentor of most economic measures that have been adopted since Second World War. Yet the celebrated economist was a maverick of his time, and had difficulty publishing his book that offered path-breaking ideas. He advocated budget deficits in bad times but surplus budgets in good times, so that the government could balance its books over the course of the business cycle. What he denounced was the balancing of the budget every year, because it required raising taxes during a recession, where the tax revenue inevitably falls. But now the governments borrow during good and bad times, something that must be disturbing Keynes in his grave. I suspect, if he was alive today, he would be in favour of devising an anchor, may it be gold, silver or both, tied to the currency in circulation. I suspect he would also recognise currency to be analogous to blood circulating in a living organism.

Keynes was guided more by common sense than the economic ideology dominant during the 1920s and the 1930s. Another luminary economist, Adam Smith, commonly known as the father of economics, also vehemently opposed contemporary views. He championed business interests based on an understanding of human nature. He exalted market competition as a force that produces a great economy, and contradicted the ideas of his peers who favoured interests of the state.

Economics, contrary to the popular belief, has ancient history. In the West, specifically Greece, it was first propounded by the likes of Plato and Aristotle. In India, it was offered by Kautilya, also known as Chanakya, who was a near contemporary of ancient Greek philosophers. Kautilya was an erudite scholar as well as a politician, who is often compared to Machiavelli, but unlike the Italian he practised politics to get rid of the oppressive rulers of his time. Thus, good economic ideas have almost always come from the works of either non-economists or maverick economists, who were often denounced by their peers.

As I said earlier, I am not an economist by profession, but I believe I have more than required common sense. And the way our economy is working today suggests that markets have multiple personalities, where valuations are out of control and extreme volatility prevails. The ideas I offer are based on the long experience of a real estate businessman, market trader as well as an engineer who knows how important it is to maintain a balance among opposing forces to create a stable machine or structure. I also have a good understanding of human nature and have written a book and articles about it. Ultimately, an ideal economy must be linked to a thorough analysis of what *homo sapiens* are, how they think and react, and what makes them happy. Contemporary economic ideas, in my view, derive from a one-sided view of human nature, namely that greed is natural, widespread and ultimately good for the people and our system. While greed can neither be ignored nor suppressed, it is not the only cog in human nature. There are many other qualities that describe our behaviour. The current economic imbalance, in the end, relates to a faulty view of what people really are. Here, in brief, is what you should expect from this book.

To begin with, the idea of a good economy is intertwined with the question of ethics, but ethical concepts have changed over time. What was ethical yesterday may be considered unethical today. Many well-meaning scholars in the past regarded slavery as part of a natural order; they thought that some people were just born in bondage and there was nothing anyone could do about it. Even Plato and Aristotle considered slavery to be natural. But we know that the practice was immoral then, as now. What was regarded as natural in the past is considered a heinous institution today. So the question relating to a good economy is this: Should an ideal economy be based on universal and time-invariant ethical standards or should it be linked to relative ethics that vary with time and space? Please note that there is no such thing as an absolute or "absolutely unchanging" in Nature, since experience tells us that everything will change sooner or later. I believe that a good economy should incorporate as many universal ethical norms as possible, and very few relative ethical norms. A well-known ethical principle is: do unto others what you would have others do unto you. This perhaps is the best moral imperative of all time, and is universally accepted. It is easily understood as everyone can relate to it; it represents time-invariant ethics, and an ideal economy ought to have institutions that are linked to this idea.

Take, for instance, the question of unemployment

compensation, which came into being in the United States during the Great Depression. Even high-growth nations like India and much of the developing world still lack this. Some scholars don't like the idea at all, because they think it encourages workers to become lazy and live on government dole. Others denounce it as government intervention in a free economy that may prolong unemployment. We will examine such ideological arguments in a later chapter. For now, let's explore their ethical content.

When a person is laid off, for no fault of his own, then it is only fair that the state should provide his family some assistance until he finds another job. Of course, the assistance should not be overly generous, or else the fired worker could find joblessness to his liking. However, classical economists, the predecessors of Keynes, were staunchly opposed to any idea that gave comfort to a labourer, whom they regarded as inherently lethargic and unwilling to work except under the pressure of hunger. Some scholars still support this view, but put yourself in the position of a jobless person. Would you want a helping hand from the government if you are fired in spite of your hard work and merit? If you say "yes", then temporary unemployment compensation should be offered in any ideal economy. In fact, most advanced economies offer this insurance today. Switzerland was the first to introduce it as early as 1789; in Britain it appeared in 1911, but other wealthy nations legislated it during the 1930s.

Thus the age-old proverb — do unto others what you would have others do unto you — can serve as a simple yet potent guideline for a good economic system. Similarly, we can say that production and commerce are good and beneficial, but intentionally helping yourselves at the expense of others is not acceptable.

What about relative ethics? Some people argue that morality varies among nations, cultures and even religions.

What is morally acceptable at one place may not be acceptable at another. What works here may not work over there. Take, for instance, the US minimum wage legislation, which was also the product of the Great Depression, and is more controversial than any other legislation born during that crisis. Many argue that the minimum wage generates unemployment especially among teenagers and does more harm than good. Others, like libertarians, denounce it as an unwarranted intrusion in a free-market system. Regardless of this ideological opposition, the minimum wage today is an important part of advanced economies. This is one area where the absolute and the relative ethical principles can conflict. The idea of the minimum wage seems to be morally right, but if it leads to joblessness then its benefit is dubious. Similarly, an appropriate minimum wage in America may be overly burdensome to the employer in India. So here what is good for one nation may be wrong for another. An ideal economy must tackle the choice between universal and relative ethics, and I shall do this in the pages to come. However, as much as possible, the economy should be based on widespread ethical standards so that poverty is removed from all nations. One thing is for sure: every nation should have a safety net that provides food to everyone; no one should go hungry. I recall an Indian proverb. "All ten virtues will disappear in the face of hunger."

Economic Trade-Offs

The idea of a trade-off, which is central to economic theory, refers to the fact that one cannot obtain something good without giving up something useful. Some people call it the cost-benefit analysis, that is, every benefit has some cost. At the level of individual behaviour, the validity of the idea is obvious, but for the economy as a whole, its application may be dubious. This is also a question that must be tackled in a treatise on the ideal economy.

There are many well-known trade-offs in economics, the most famous being the inflation-unemployment trade-off, which, having been named after R.J.W. Phillips, an academic from London School of Economics, is also called the Phillips Curve. The theory is that low unemployment requires a higher rate of inflation, and conversely. Both rising prices and joblessness are evil, and we have to choose between the two. This theme, which was very popular in the 1960s and early 1970s, died in the next two decades, and seemed to make a comeback at the end of the 2000s. It has had its ups and downs, and Mr. Bernanke seems to have revived it by injecting billions of dollars of new money into the economy. The proponents of the inflation-unemployment trade-off have one ready answer for every problem: When in trouble, print more money. If it leads to higher inflation, so be it, because joblessness is a worse evil than soaring prices. The trade-off advocates thus have an absolutist view of ethics — namely recessions should be avoided at all cost. However, there are times when a recession may be just what the doctor ordered.

During the 1970s, the Fed chairmen followed what Mr. Bernanke is doing now. They printed more money every time the oil price went up, mostly to avoid rising unemployment. They wanted to restrain a rise in the interest rate to stimulate the housing market and thus the economy, which is also the objective of the current Fed chairman. But repeated injections of money into the economy gave rise to horrendous inflation by the end of the 1970s, and ironically interest rates shot up to unprecedented levels. This was the unintended consequence of monetary injections. The housing market then collapsed, cars went unsold, and the United States, along with the world, suffered the worst recession since Second World War. So, at times, relative ethics may be superior to absolute ethics. Avoiding recession at all cost is an absolute ethical norm, whereas permitting recession to fight inflation requires a belief in relative ethics, which is in fact, what Paul Volcker, the Fed chairman in the early 1980s, did. He reversed the policy of ever higher monetary stimulus to combat unemployment; interest rates soared even more, the recession worsened, but inflation cooled significantly and laid the foundation of subsequent economic revival.

A well-known Austrian-American economist, Joseph Schumpeter, invented the idea of what is known as "creative destruction", wherein firms fail and workers are fired only to lead to the birth of new and efficient businesses that hire those fired workers and are able to pay higher wages because of improving productivity. Such tumult is regarded as an integral part of the evolution of capitalism, wherein markets function to reward talent and penalise mistakes. What Volcker did was something akin to Schumpeter's preaching, except that he intentionally raised interest rates to deepen the slump to get rid of soaring prices. In the process, he took a lot of heat from politicians who by instinct fear recessions, but historians have been very kind to him. Economists then recognised the futility of the inflation-employment trade-off, but it appears that Mr. Bernanke has to learn the lessons of ignoring inflation anew. He bailed out Bear Stearns and injected bushels of money into the banking system for the greater good of society, but set a bad precedent that could come back to haunt him in the guise of high inflation.

According to Schumpeter, even "Depressions are not simply evils which we might attempt to suppress", as, "they represent something that has to be done". Others like Brad DeLong, an economic historian at the University of California, Berkeley, reinforce Schumpeter's callous logic by arguing that recessions help release resources from profitless activities into productive areas and thus enhance the living standard in the long run. *The Economist* echoes the same theme: "One could think of the recession similar to pruning the tree." This line of reasoning gives rise to an interesting question: Do we need creative destruction in an ideal economy? Is it necessary to put the system into violent spasms to accelerate the rise in living standards? It is true that ups and downs are part of nature, but do they have to be violent? This is another issue tackled by this work.

Another well-known idea in economics refers to the equity-efficiency trade-off, popularised by Arthur Okun. Okun suggested that an egalitarian economy generates a lower level of economic growth and efficiency. Therefore, society has to make a choice between equity and efficiency, because lower inequality means a lower living standard for people. This theory is supported by the CEOs, because it offers a simple justification for their incredible wealth and salaries. Many analysts, economists and others hired by the CEOs, also believe in it, but on its face it seems to be a self-serving logic. Yet this trade-off can be found in almost every textbook on economics.

Some scholars argue that higher growth produces higher pollution, and the recent experience of India and China tends to confirm this view. There is then a trade-off between growth and the environment. However, the Japanese experience with economic development is different, because there the rising living standards since 1970 has not generated increased pollution. Thus, the growth-pollution trade-off may also be dubious.

This book argues that an ideal economy ought not to face such contradictions. There are and always will be trade-offs at the individual level, but proper economic policy can help societies avoid them. It is not necessary that at the macro level we have to give up something useful to obtain something good, at least in terms of inflation *versus* unemployment, or equity *versus* efficiency. It should be possible to eliminate both high joblessness and inflation at the same time or to create an efficient, high-growth economy without generating higher inequality.

Human Nature

It should be obvious that an ideal economy must be linked to human nature. If not, the system will fall apart sooner rather than later. But what exactly is human nature? Even though the concept is obvious to most of us, there are disagreements over it among various schools of thought. We would all concur that people want to be happy, and their actions are motivated mostly by thoughts of pleasure and pain. But what makes people happy is open to question.

"Man", said Aristotle, "is, by nature, a social animal", which essentially means that man has animalistic needs and tendencies, and that he likes to live in groups to survive, thrive and be happy. He seeks to form a family, which may be large or small. It may be a family of just two or many more. It is well known that family people live longer and are healthier. So there is a large grain of truth in Aristotle's celebrated statement, but it is partial and does not fully describe what or who we really are. Man is much more than an animal.[1]

Like other creatures, we do have physical needs, but we also are emotional and self-reflecting. Interaction with others is much valued, but so is privacy. We like to dwell in groups and society, but at times we want to be left alone, and contemplate our origins and a deeper meaning of life. In common parlance, we have bodies, minds and souls, or as I like to say, human being has three selves — the somatic self, the psychic self and the spiritual self.

A close examination reveals that the human personality has three domains within it, each one equal and autonomous. This is the crucial point that the three ingredients of the human self are independent of each other and are equally important. None can be neglected for the sake of happiness. The somatic self, consists of the body and genetics; the psychic self, consists of intuition and intellect; and the spiritual self is at the centre of the other two.

The somatic self, the domain of primal urges and energies, is where the DNA comes into play. It deals with health, vigour and stamina. Even though independent, it is closely connected to the psychic self, which itself has two aspects — the intellect and the intuition. The intellect relates to reason and logic or the lack thereof, whereas the intuition reflects a person's gentler emotions such as love, compassion and forgiveness. The spiritual self is the same as the soul.

A person may have a poor intellect but a rich intuition. Conversely, a person may be very smart yet brutal. According to ancient Indian sages, who composed the Vedas and Vedanta, a developed total human self, with intellect and intuition in balance and harmony, is the only gateway to the spiritual self. "Veda" means "to know", and "Vedanta" signifies "the end or culmination of knowledge". The sages suggested that a human self, in balance with full control over senses and a rich intuition, transports itself from the realm of the finite to that of the infinite, from the knowable to something beyond human comprehension.

There is no limit to the desires and greed of the body. Man must meet certain basic needs or perish. He must eat, drink, sleep, remain healthy and procreate not just to perpetuate the human species but also to satisfy a powerful instinct. There seems to be no end to his wants, wishes and requirements. His needs, according to the Western tradition, constitute man's innate nature. But the Vedic tradition holds that such needs reflect only a part of human nature. There are two other selves as well, and they are autonomous and equally important for happiness.

Nirmal Kumar, a prominent Indian philosopher-psychologist, offers a clear-cut view of what the Vedas describe as the psychic self, which in most people identifies itself with the somatic self. Most people think of themselves as their bodies; they ascribe their actions and feelings to their brains. Ask someone who he is; he will point his thumb towards his chest and say, "My name is this and I am such and such a person". In fact, people are too afraid to think of themselves as different from their bodies. They cannot even imagine their existence without the somatic self. However, the Vedas say that your body is not you but something similar to a garment. When a person develops a much higher state of mind, and can disassociate himself from his somatic self, he transcends the realm of physicality and comes to the doorsteps of the spiritual self. He frees himself from somatic limitations and their pain. He becomes joyous and ever blissful. Such is the goal of human life, as presented by the Vedas and the Vedanta.

The Vedas also tell us that man is part of Nature, like all other creatures. Nature lies within us, just like the spiritual self and should not be violated. We have to live in accordance with our surroundings and not destroy them. Thus, happiness arises when man lives in harmony with Nature, and leads a life of balance among the three selves. Other thinkers suggest that man is a social but greedy animal. Animals are mostly satisfied with their possessions, but man wants more and more. He never seems to be content with what he has and seeks to accumulate wealth beyond his needs. Adam Smith, a British economist and philosopher, emphasised this human trait in his 1776 masterpiece, *The Wealth of Nations*, and used it to build a whole new approach to economics. He argued that a good economy is one that works with man's self-centred nature rather than suppresses it through government edicts. He suggested that greed should not be condemned but tolerated, because it creates an efficient economy through the principle of what he called, "the invisible hand of the market". He championed tough competition among firms to create free enterprise and denounced state monopolies that bulged large in his day. Ever since Smith's path-breaking work, "greed is good" has become the main *mantra* of capitalism, even though the system has become far more monopolistic than that envisioned by him.

Aristotle's social animal, Smith's greedy creature and the three selves of the Vedas can be combined to get a true picture of human nature. The Western tradition can be blended with ancient Indian thought to comprehend what truly brings us happiness. Briefly speaking, in my view, happiness occurs when a family person lives in a truly free-market economy and leads a life that is harmonious with Nature and his three selves.

One prerequisite of an ideal economy, as stated above, is that it must conform to human nature or else disintegrate. What all this suggests is that a good economic system is one that enables people to pursue happiness from an amiable family life and by attending to their three selves. When people have enough time not only to make a good living but also to cater to the well-being of their children and engage in achieving higher mental states, then they have an ever rising joyous life. They should not have to spend much of their time to make both ends meet.

Let us consider a typical family of four — husband, wife and two children. Until the end of the 1960s, one family person, mainly the husband, could earn enough in the United States to support the entire family adequately, i.e. buy a home, a car, feed the children, send them to neighbourhood schools, and take good care of their health. When the children came back from school, they would fall into the loving arms of their mother, who would also help them with their homework, impart ethical values, and offer them freshly cooked food. This was the American dream, but it was also a dream cherished around the world. It was also accessible to people in Canada, much of Europe and Australia. The system was such that it offered a good family life as well as time for prayer. People could also spare hours and go to a temple, mosque or church for solace. Thus, the post-Second World War era up until 1970 offered an economy tending towards perfection in the United States. Please note that the research done by Professor R. Barro and R. McCleary of Harvard University confirms that the belief in God is good for economic growth (*The Economist*, 15 November 2003).

The American dream began to evaporate in the 1970s and is turning into a nightmare at the end of the 2000s. Obviously something has gone awry in the past 40 years. Today families are harried and breaking down. The real wage, or the purchasing power of a person's salary, is insufficient to support a typical family, which requires two adults to labour outside their home. Working hours and tension have also multiplied. According to an eminent Indian scholar, Deepak Chopra, Americans die mostly from stress, not disease. Job dissatisfaction, not illness, is the largest killer of people in America. He proves his point by showing that most heart attacks occur on Monday morning at 9. It is the first day of the work week, and many people are simply terrified to begin their stressful or unhappy work.

With two-worker families, children come home from school and find themselves in the indifferent or hostile arms of babysitters, who themselves have no clues about ethical values. Obesity is a growing problem. Lacking freshly made food at home, children munch on the offerings of McDonald's or Burger King. They are a lot heavier than before, and even Santa is afraid to hold them in his lap around Christmas. Even American youngsters now face the hazards of diabetes and heart disease.

As regards the housing market, it actually faces double jeopardy. On the one hand, homes have become so expensive that a lot of two-earner families cannot afford to buy them.

The households can't even make a down payment. On the other hand, home prices have been falling since 2007 and seem to see no bottom. Such a deadly combination of dropping family values along with unaffordable housing is unprecedented in US history. Even the mega-inflationary 1970s had better home values to offer.

In addition to housing's double jeopardy, gasoline price has been soaring since 2004. Fannie Mae and Freddie Mac have been nationalised in America, a capitalist country and a strong advocate of free enterprise! Several small airlines have declared bankruptcy while many others including the behemoths like American Airlines and United Airlines are deeply in debt. It should be clear that we no longer have an ideal economy in the United States, and, for that matter, around the globe. This is because what is happening in America is also being replicated around the world. It is indeed depressing to see the four pillars of the American economy, namely auto, housing, banking and finance, and retailing, getting weaker by the day.

The Coming Chapters

By now, my brief discussion of disparate concepts should give you an idea of what this work is all about. I see problems galore; they are appearing in droves and we need an ideal economy to eradicate them for a long time.

My next chapter examines the current mess that we find ourselves in and on how we got here in our global economy. It focuses on US history as well as the role of Japan, China, India, the European Union among others. Chapter 3 explores the good-economy concepts that we have inherited from past writings, and then focuses on what an ideal economy is like. Here I collate the views of Western and non-Western writers, especially the mavericks who almost always offer original thinking. The ideas of Kautilya, Plato, Aristotle, Ibn Khaldun,

Adam Smith, Karl Marx, the Mercantilists, the Physiocrats, Keynes, Schumpeter, contemporary Ivy-League economists, the Nobel Prize winners, and finally the controversial author and today's maverick economist, Ravi Batra, are explored in some depth. We live in a global village, and the one basic theme underlying our world is that no single culture or nation has a monopoly over good ideas. We have to collect the best views of all writers to come up with an ideal system that conforms to human nature and that will work everywhere with minor modifications consistent with time, place and person.

Chapter 4 looks at how the ideal economy is to be achieved; how it can materialise in a free democratic society. In chapter 5, I examine the various laws of nature that deal with balance, harmony, cohesion and complementarities in life and society. Finally, Chapter 6 offers a variety of economic reforms that should be undertaken to generate my cherished goal — an ideal economy.

Reference

1 Vedic scriptures explain that three forms of life were created by Brahma, the God of creation. They are animalistic demons, humans, and angels (*devas*). The rules of the game were that demons could transform themselves into humans if they adhere to compassion (*daya*). Humans could transform themselves into angels through charity (*daan*). The highest state of being, that is becoming selfless and desireless, is achieved by having full control over senses (*daman*). So *daya*, *daan*, and *daman* maintain the separation of three natural forms of life and the divine creator Himself.

2

Chills in a Seemingly Healthy Economy

On 11 July 2008, shares of Fannie Mae and Freddie Mac, the twin pillars of the US housing market, hit rock bottom, each down more than 90 per cent in a year, at a time the GDP had continued to expand. Wall Street was shaken; so were share markets around the world. A lot of worries pestered the investor. Could Fannie and Freddie fail, leaving the already tottering American housing market in a shambles? Are they not protected by government guarantees? Are they too big to fall?

In order to answer these questions, and to reassure the globe about the soundness of the US financial system, many government officials testified before Congress over the next few days. Prominent among them were Fed Chairman Ben Bernanke and Treasury Secretary Henry Paulson. A great drama unfolded, especially on 15 July, as Bernanke offered a sobering assessment of the economy, while President Bush, holding a press conference simultaneously, played down the negatives arising from the Fannie and Freddie plunge. He asserted:

> The bottom line is this: We're going through a tough time, but our economy has continued growing, consumers are spending, businesses are investing, exports continue increasing, and American productivity remains strong. We can have confidence in the long-term foundation of our

> economy, and I believe we will come through this challenge stronger than ever before.

Cable TV occasionally displayed Bernanke's testimony and Bush's conference at the same time. The split TV screen offered a dramatic contrast between Bernanke's long face and Bush's optimism. The chairman spoke the truth, while the president played politics, as most presidents and politicians do.

The president's view was dutifully echoed by other government officials, especially Paulson, who emphasised that the economy's long-term fundamentals were sound. That still failed to answer the burning question: why were the financial markets reeling in a seemingly healthy economy, with low unemployment and positive GDP growth? To answer this query we need to see how the economy has evolved since Second World War; we need to examine the trends that have created chills in a system that is still the largest in the world, but cannot provide a decent living standard to all its citizens.

Anyway, Fannie and Freddie shares stabilised in the coming weeks, thanks to a heavy dose of official intervention, offering virtually unlimited Federal Reserve credit to the two companies and a promise to buy their shares, if necessary. The unthinkable had happened. Imagine a George Bush government, with its heavy rhetoric of free markets, promising to buy Freddie and Fannie shares in case of another plunge. It smacks of socialism, which, coming from the Republican administration of Bush and Cheney, suggests that things must be a lot worse than what the president acknowledged in his press conference.

However, we need to realise that the seeds of some of the current economic problems were sown in the later part of the 1960s and the early 1970s. For instance, the Vietnam War along with the government's guns and butter policy, which amounted to having your cake and eating it too, led to the culture of growing budget deficits that are now exploding;

the oil embargo imposed by the Organization of Petroleum Exporting Countries (OPEC) in 1973 and the subsequent quadrupling of oil prices led to soaring inflation, from which we are now suffering again. The Watergate scandal spawned a culture of corruption that seeped into official economic policy, and so on. The moral is that the seeds of the current economic malaise were planted a long time ago and they are now producing their sour fruit.

The Immediate Post-war Economy

Second World War ended in 1945. The immediate result was a sharp decline in defence-related government spending, which spawned fears of a major recession. However, private spending shot up to make up for all the restraints that consumers had put on themselves to save more and buy government bonds during the hostilities. So no recession materialised; in fact, inflation zoomed because of soaring consumption.

Following the war, the United States emerged by far the predominant economy in the world. Its military supremacy as well as industrial might was unchallenged. Out of altruism, compassion or self-interest, the nation set out to bolster both Europe and Japan to reconstruct their shrivelled economies. The assistance came in the form of foreign aid (Marshal/ MacArthur Plans), grants, loans, open markets and new technology.

US corporations were the most competitive and productive at the time; they feared no one and were not afraid to face import competition. The dollar was a strong currency, and perhaps one reason for its strength was that it was convertible into gold at a fixed rate of $35 per ounce, so that the Federal Reserve had a restraint on its ability to print money and debase the value of our currency. However, things changed rapidly in a matter of two decades, as both Europe and Japan began to industrialise with unprecedented vigour and began to challenge the American might. At first, the import challenge came in the form of light and low-tech products such as shoes, textiles, toys, sports paraphernalia, among others; later it came from high-tech goods such as autos, tractors, televisions, robotics, electronics and optics, computers and sophisticated machine tools. European and Japanese automakers began to take a significant market share in the late 1960s.

By 1970, the fundamental character of the US economy began to change at a fast pace. Its industrial might that had mostly survived the challenge thus far began a long-term decline. Its manufacturing base began to erode, giving way to a service economy, along with minor growth of new high-tech products. Its exports began to lag behind its imports, leading to a slow but steady rise in its trade deficit. Its currency began to fall, and needed periodic intervention from central banks around the world to remain stable. In short, the wide variety of problems that the US faces today first appeared in the early 1970s in the wake of a decline in American competitiveness in world markets. The political turmoil caused by the Vietnam War and the Watergate scandal, together with the dissatisfaction of the younger generation did not help, either.

GDP and the Living Standard

We can say without any fear of contradiction that an ideal economy should produce a high and rising living standard for all; but how do we define or measure a nation's standard of living? There was little debate on this question until the early 1990s. Most economists believed that a country's aggregate output or GDP (gross domestic product) per person was the best yardstick of its general prosperity. Such was the consensus all over the world. The United Nations as well as the International Monetary Fund conducted extensive research, making international comparisons of per capita GDP.

The higher the figure, the higher the national living standard, they said. However, all this changed when Professor Ravi Batra of Southern Methodist University, USA, challenged this view in his 1993 work, *The Myth of Free Trade*.

Even now the majority of economists, including Robert Barro, Robert Lucas, Alan Greenspan and Ben Bernanke, hold per capita GDP as the main, if not the only, gauge of society's well-being. Since per capita GDP is the nation's output per person, on its face the popular viewpoint seems eminently plausible. Society, after all, is the sum total of its people, and their aggregate output ought to indicate their level of consumption and hence material happiness. The more you produce and consume, the bigger is your level of comfort. If you can afford better cars, food, education, housing and health care, there is no doubt you are materially better off than before.

Batra argues further that the distribution of GDP among individuals matters just as much as its size. If this distribution becomes more and more unequal over time, then per capita GDP may be a deceptive indicator of social well-being. It is well known that a nation's output also approximates its aggregate income, which in turn is divided among the people. Suppose 60 per cent of the people suffer a wage decline, is it possible for the aggregate income and hence GDP to rise? The answer is "yes", provided the incomes of the 40 per cent rise more than the total for the other 60 per cent. In this case, the general living standard has declined because the majority is worse off than before, even though per capita GDP goes up.

Batra went on to argue that such a case was not just a theoretical possibility but an actual description of the American economy since the early 1970s. He proposed an alternative measure of the living standard and called it the production wage. According to the BLS (Bureau of Labor Statistics), a US government agency, workers may be divided into two categories — supervisory workers and the non-supervisory workers, who are also called production workers, i.e. those that work under the supervision of others. The average real wage of the production worker may be called the production wage, which, according to Batra, is the best measure of the living standard, because it applies to at least 75 per cent of the workforce. The term "real" indicates purchasing power. So the production wage measures the purchasing power of the average salary earned by non-supervisory workers. It separates the production worker from the managerial worker, and excludes capital income that is at the root of the growing income disparity.

Subsequent to Batra's contribution, others such as MIT economist Lester Thurow, Harvard law professor Elizabeth Warren and her daughter Amelia Warren Tyagi, best-selling author Thom Hartmann, and Economic Policy Institute economists Lawrence Mishel and Jared Bernstein also discarded GDP as a good measure of society's well-being. Instead, they examined real family income, which takes into account the wages of all family members, and concluded that the average American worker was overworked and suffered a fall in the comfort level or living standard, because even though the family income continued to rise in spite of the falling wage, family expenses rose even faster and showed up in the sinking savings rate. Numerous books have appeared in recent years to document the decimation of the American middle class. None of them accepts per capita GDP as an accurate measure of the living **standard.**[1]

The Production Wage and Family Income

Let us explore the behaviour of the production wage and family income in America since 1950. A readable and fairly comprehensive statistical book called the *Economic Report of the President* (*ERP*) is published every year by the government. This is a compendium of widely used figures, and offers data on both family income and the production wage. This data is presented in *fig.* 1 at five-year intervals to smooth out short-term fluctuations. Since the period under consideration is long, smoothing out the data simply aids our comprehension. Another modification has been done to the family income data by dividing it by 100 and thus converting it into an index. This has been done to present it along with real weekly earnings in the same graph, because ultimately we seek an easy way to see the trends in the two variables.

The figure shows something very interesting. The production wage went up steadily from 1950 to 1973, and then began a long-term decline. It was $331 per week in 1973 and $281 in 2007. Real family income, by contrast, offers a different trend. It also rose steadily from 1950 to 1973, fell a little that year because of a recession but then resumed its upward march from 1975 till 1990, fell again until 1995, resumed its rise, peaked in 2000, and then began to fall even after the recession of 2001 which ended in 2002. It crested at $63,189 in

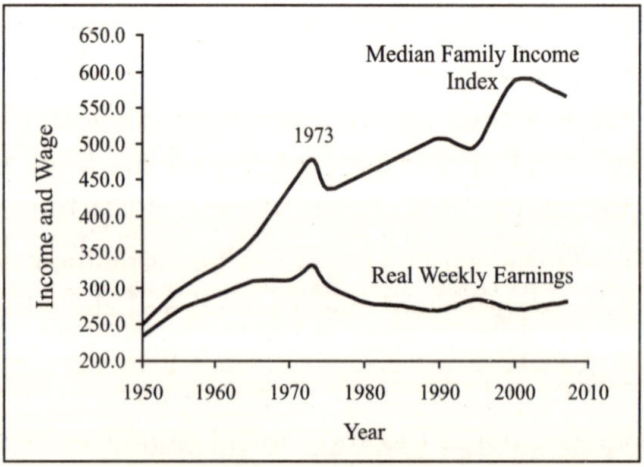

fig 1: Production Wage and Family Income in the US 1950-2007

Source: The *ERP*, various years. Weekly earnings are in terms of 1982 dollars, and median family income in terms of 2006 dollars. This is the way *ERP*, 2008, presents the data, and some figures from 1950 to 1990 were taken from other *ERP*s and adjusted for base year changes.

2000, according to the 2011 *ERP* and had decreased by more than $3,000 by 2009. Thus the production wage never recovered the height of 1973, and family income that used to fall only during recessions in the past is still way below its peak.

Fig. 2 displays the behaviour of per capita GDP and labour productivity, both of which reveal a general upward trend, which is somewhat shocking, because it suggests that while the vast majority of Americans have been getting more and more productive, their wage and now household incomes have been falling. In other words, the overall economy is doing well except for the people in it. The behaviour of per capita GDP indicates that the US living standard has been rising ever since the war, but the production wage and even family income offer a conflicting testimony. What has happened is that about a quarter of the population has gained so much that the overall economy shows positive growth even though the other three quarter of the people has suffered a declining standard of living.

The production wage indicates a living standard loss since 1973, whereas the family income data suggests a decline since 2001. Which of the two views is correct? It appears to me that the production wage is a better indicator than the family income measure, simply because when both members of a household work outside their home, then children must suffer, and that suffering is rarely quantified. It may be interesting to look into the statistical data on matters of education quality in public schools, crime rate among the younger population, drug use, children born out of wedlock and so on. In all these respects, we are worse off today than in the 1970s. The prison population, for instance, jumped by 700 per cent between 1970 and 2005. Almost half of the increase was due to expanding drug use among the **youth**.[2] It is also well known that the American high-school education has been on a long-term decline. There is now even a documentary called "Two Million

Minutes" to demonstrate this trend. The film shows Americans generally having fun socialising and playing games while foreign students spend hours mastering algebra and arithmetic.

Much of this change can be attributed to the rise of the two-worker families that tend to slight the homemaker's contribution to the development of children. Several studies have shown that the market value of the unpaid household work done by a homemaker is quite large, ranging from $30,000 to $90,000 per **year,**[3] **and** if that value is subtracted from median family income to obtain the net income from the second worker's job, the resulting figure would not show much gain, and could show a loss. In any case, once again it is clear that the US is far from an ideal system today.

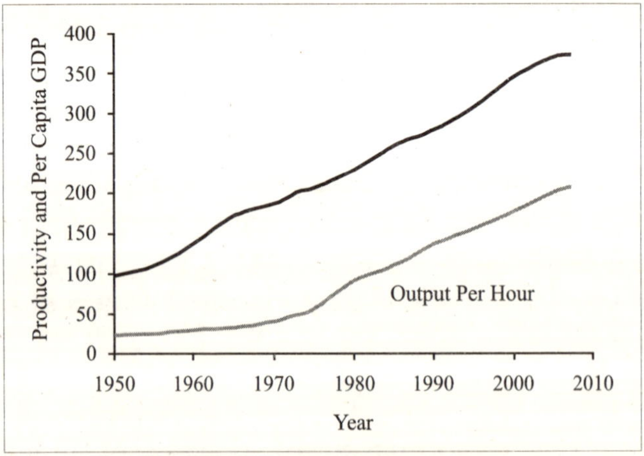

fig. 2: Per capita GDP and Productivity in the United States: 1950-2007

Source: The *ERP*, various years. Output per hour is in terms of 1992 dollars, and per capita GDP in terms of 2000 dollars.

Nature and the Law of Balancing the Opposites

When a non-economist approaches economics, he is struck by the multiplicity of theories, especially in macroeconomics, the one dealing with society's well-being. All of the theories seem to make sense, but we know that some would have greater validity than the others. They all cannot have the same weight; normally, one of them would be closest to the truth, given that the truth here refers to a rise in the living standard of all the people. The truth in Eastern traditions is analogous to facets of a cut and polished diamond. Each facet is pretty to look at but only one is the largest and the prettiest. In other words, one of the macroeconomic theories should be able to explain how the economy truly works so as to make everyone comfortable, and then how to solve our problems. However, there are numerous schools of economic thought. They include classicists, Keynesians, neo-classicists, neo-Keynesians, monetarists, supply-siders, libertarians, mercantilists, socialists, communists, free traders, protectionists, and on and on.

Even among economists within a school there is seldom agreement; what should a non-economist then do? Of course, he can resort to common sense, but all economists claim that they make sense. Before we turn to technical theories in the coming chapters, let me note that there is another way out of this dilemma, and that is to look to the universally acclaimed natural law of balancing the opposites to survive and prosper. Although here we are talking more of philosophy than of modern economics, it may be noted that many prominent economists, including Adam Smith, were also philosophers. Philosophy sometimes provides answers to the questions that elude the experts.

The law of balancing the opposites says that almost everything in Nature has two opposing sides that must be balanced in order to find peace, vigour, and harmony in life.

Also known as the principle of polarity, this law suggests that virtually everything has two sides, two poles, two aspects. They are just a pair of opposites, with various degrees of expression between extremes. Such polarity is so pervasive that it is nearly impossible to describe the quality of any entity without referring to its other side. This is because everything is relative in this world. Something is hot only because something else is cold. There are manifold degrees of heat and chillness, but one cannot exist without the other.

Thus good and evil, life and death, knowledge and ignorance, pleasure and pain, gain and loss are just like two sides of the same coin. In fact, the Eastern traditions believe that good and evil are the same as knowledge and ignorance and cannot be separated. The process of education becomes the bridge to mitigate and overcome problems associated with ignorance. The organisms and organisations must be in balance and in harmony within, and they must learn to live close to the centre of the multi-dimensional space of their existence. The boundary or extremity of this space is not a fine line of demarcation but a cluster of rising barriers, where the black swan, to use a phrase coined by Nassim Taleb in his book with the same title, thrives. The phrase refers to a large and unpredictable impact from events that occur in extremities of the standard bell curve. Taleb calls them Extremistan as opposed to Mediocristan where predictability increases. Examples of black swans include the 9/11 episode, the 2005 and 2011 tsunamis and the rise of the Internet, i.e. rare events beyond the realm of normal expectations. Extremistan seems to be a venue for both the birth of a new order and/or the death of an old order; in terms of Hindu mythology, these orders are of great significance where the god of creation, Brahma, and the god of destruction, Shiva, are active. Mediocristan seems to be a venue for routine existence and mediocrity where the god of sustenance, Vishnu, is active.

Extremistan is not necessarily "Chaostan" but a place where rare and monumental events take place; these events may generate chaos, destruction, or new systems. There is always an attempt by scholars to make the black swan event predictable after it has occurred, which to my mind has little value.

The pairs of opposites are so pervasive that one might say that it is Nature's favourite sport to create them for the purpose of their mutual survival. Living organisms coexist in multidimensional space to survive. Multiple pairs of opposites constitute multidimensional space. In an unpredictable Nature, these multiple pairs must exist to maintain life. Elements of a pair of opposites cannot be separated, any more than the north pole of a magnet can be separated from the south pole. Ancient Vedic teachers would say that the opposites need to complement each other, instead of competing or remaining at war so that they can complement, coexist in balance and harmony to survive and prosper. Philosophers like Hegel and psychologists such as Jung have also used the law of balancing the opposites in their work.

Furthermore, the organisms and organisations must stay at locations away from multiple boundaries, because they may perish if they hit a boundary. It is safest to be in the centre of a multidimensional space, although it may not be as rewarding as being in the centre. A zebra remaining in the centre of the herd is probably safest from an attack by a predator; however, this animal may not have access to the freshest grass. A presidential candidate almost always claims the centre to increase the likelihood of getting elected. His defeat becomes more likely if he holds either the ultra-leftist or ultra-rightist views. Barry Goldwater's failure in the 1964 presidential race, and George McGovern's in 1972 are just two examples of how extremism does not work in an election. Please note that the location of the centre is never absolute in nature; it is relative and depends upon many variables, including mass psychology of the population. Nature makes the centre and extremes of the multidimensional space relative and changing. Senator Goldwater's statement that "extremism in the defence of the country is no vice, and the pursuit of moderation is no virtue" was rejected in 1964. However, a resounding majority accepted this notion in a nation hurt by the 9/11 massacre. The laws of evolution and change apply to all domains of our existence.

The laws governing the pairs of opposites by themselves would perhaps have little significance for us, except that they offer a valuable lesson, namely if the opposites move too far away creating large imbalance, there is trouble, sometimes calamity. Take, for instance, a tornado, which arises when extremely cold air collides with extremely hot air, leading to destruction of life and property.

According to ancient sages, opposites are two sides of the same reality and are ultimately the expressions of one and the same entity. Since they represent the same entity, there should be balance and harmony between them rather than perpetual conflict. The Chinese philosophers refer to the dynamic interplay of two extremes as Ying and Yang (positive and negative). Hindu God Shiva is often represented as half man and half woman to show the balance and completeness of being. Science looks at the opposing sides as positively and negatively charged particles of matter, which combine to generate a natural reaction. A tornado is a natural reaction of a kind. It could be avoided if there is a broad path of diffusion.

An analogous argument can be made for economics, which also deals with numerous pairs of opposites that must be closely balanced to generate a vigorous and healthy economy. In foreign trade, for instance, exports are a complement to imports; in the federal budget, spending is on the opposite side of tax revenue; in the domestic economy, investment cannot exist without savings, borrowers cannot exist without lenders. In the labour market, the real wage and labour productivity are merely the two sides of the same coin called production. These opposites are quantifiable and hence not subject to multiple interpretations. That is what is good about economics. Since every economic phenomenon is subject to measurement, there should be one theory capable of explaining their cause. This will be examined in detail in Chapter 5.

Balancing the Pairs of Economic Opposites

The law of balancing the opposites implies that a sound economic system requires the economic pairs of opposites to complement each other and not compete or be at war. They should not be far apart or hit their boundaries. Thus, the demand for anything should be close to its supply, otherwise profits will suffer and production will decline. We have seen that the immediate post-war economy in the US was very healthy. At that time, the real wage went up with productivity, one family member could provide decent lifestyle to a household of four, consumer debt was small, and the living standard rose for all. It turns out that the 1950s and the 1960s were also the decades when the economic pairs of opposites were in close balance to each other.

Government spending and tax revenue were more or less the same in the federal budget. The budget deficit was either zero or miniscule. Family discretionary income on the average was much higher than what it is today. But see what happened over time in *fig*. 3 under various administrations. The figure deals with two variables, the budget and the trade deficit as a percentage of GDP during the tenure of nine presidencies following Second World War. The budget shortfall or surplus is cumulative for each administration, that is, it is the sum total of the annual deficit to GDP ratio during a presidency.

Under President Truman, the budget was actually in a small surplus, about 0.2 per cent of GDP, and turned into a deficit under the administrations of Eisenhower, Kennedy and Johnson. However, the deficit was still rather small, around 1 per cent of the GDP. Budgetary red ink began to rise with Nixon and Ford, stabilised under Carter and then soared from Reagan on. It fell under President Clinton — in fact, the budget turned into a surplus towards the end of Clinton's second term — but then made a resounding comeback under President Bush II. The administration's latest projection in mid-2008 put the 2009 deficit at $482 billion, which would be an all-time high in absolute number, although in percentage terms no president has beaten the annual record set by President Reagan at 6 per cent. The crux of the matter is that the budget deficit was extremely low during the 1950s and the 1960s, and rose steadily and sharply during the 1970s, 1980s and the 2000s. President Clinton provided the only exception to US budget fiascos.

A similar fate awaited foreign commerce. The trade deficit in *fig*. 3 is the balance on goods and services and is not cumulative for each presidency; rather, in view of the available data, it reflects the deficit as a per cent of GDP at the end of each term. During the 1950s and 1960s, under Truman, Eisenhower, Kennedy and Johnson, the US had a closer balance in trade, with a small surplus. In fact, the trade surplus lasted longer than the initial budget surplus. Then came the 1970s, and at the end of Nixon-Ford presidency in 1976, the surplus turned into a small deficit, only to zoom during the 1980s and beyond. The Yom Kippur War and the oil embargo in 1973 by the OPEC added fuel to the fire.

Some scholars see a cause-and-effect scenario in terms of *fig*. 3, arguing that high budget deficits lead to high trade shortfall. Here the cause-and-effect link is at best, tenuous. It is true that as the budgetary red ink went up from 1970 to 1990, the trade deficit also rose; but then the budget deficit

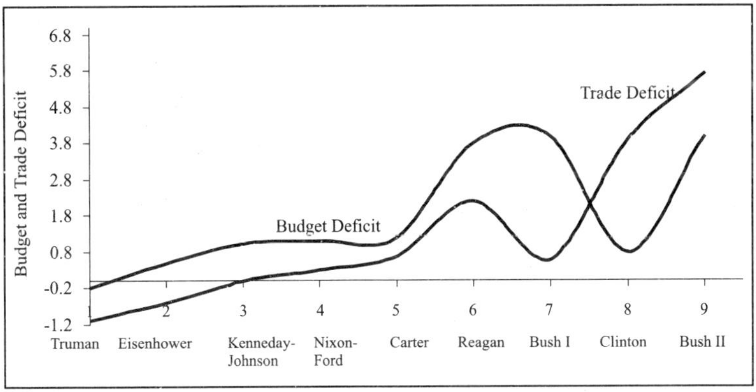

fig. 3: The Trade and Budget Deficit as a per cent of GDP under Various Presidents since Second World War

Source: The *ERP*, various years

rose sharply under Bush I and the trade shortfall declined, whereas the opposite happened under Clinton. However, under Bush II, both deficits rocketed, thanks to the 9/11 terror attack and the wars in Iraq and Afghanistan, and then continued to rise at a dizzying pace under President Obama.

With the rise in the budget deficit, the government's debt, which is the cumulative total of the annual deficit, had to rise. This is documented in *fig.* 4, which shows that at first national debt as a percentage of GDP experienced a long-term decline after 1950. The reason is that during the war the government was forced to borrow a lot of money to fight Hitler and Japan; so its debt soared. After the war defence spending plummeted, the budget moved into surplus for a while, war debt was slowly retired, and as GDP rose the ratio of debt to GDP had to fall. The ratio kept falling for a time even when the budget deficit started to rise from Eisenhower (Ike) on, because the GDP growth was very strong. As a matter of fact, the debt ratio fell until Carter, and then began to rise furiously under Reagan and later, under Bush II.

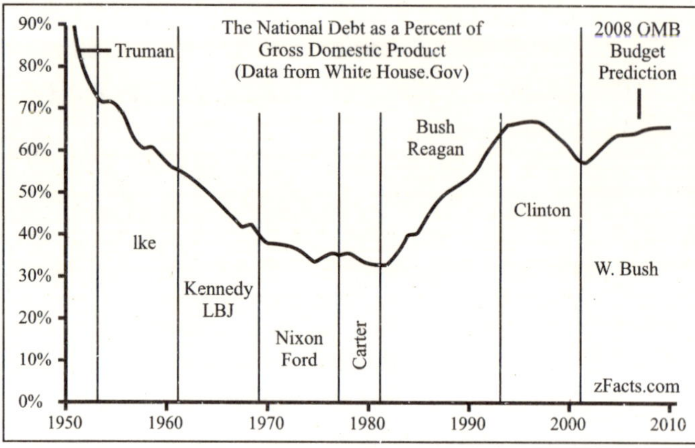

Fig. 4: National Debt since Second World War
Source: zfacts.com, and
The *ERP*, various years.

The national debt has simply skyrocketed since 1980. It is now well known that the cumulative debt generated by all 39 presidents prior to Reagan was a bit shy of $1 trillion. By the end of Reagan's presidency, however, it had shot up to over $2.6 trillion. President Reagan was a superman. He alone did to the national red ink what all other presidents before him could not do. However, Bush II went a step further. If Reagan's debt contribution was $1.7 trillion, Bush II's exceeded $4 trillion. Thus the jump in national debt has been fast and furious, and has resulted from violating Nature's law that calls for balancing the pairs of opposites. The Reagan-Bush economic policies brought inflation under control and may have many other merits, but they certainly left a heavy burden on the shoulders of our children who will have to deal with consequences of the red ink. But the red ink often occurred in a divided government with the two parties either controlling the legislature or the executive branch, but rarely both branches. Thus, the Democrats held a majority in the House of Representatives in the early 1980s when Reagan was president. Under Bush I both Houses were under Democratic control, whereas under Clinton, both Houses for a while came under Republican control.

How are the twin debts, domestic and foreign, linked to the imbalance of the opposites? In the case of the budget deficit, the opposites are clear; they are government spending and revenue, and the deficit is the difference between them. These opposites have been moving away from each other, generating a growing pile of national debt. If the transition to lower taxes and lower government spending was necessary, it should have been done with much smaller increase in the deficit.

The trade deficit occurs when the two opposites, exports and imports, move apart from each other. As imports exceed exports, there is trade shortfall, and someone has to finance it. Either we pay for it in terms of gold, or the foreign country must be ready to accept our currency. We are not exporting our gold to other nations, who are content to accept the payment in terms of our paper dollars. Their dollar horde adds annually to our obligations. This way, we borrow money from them and they are in a position to buy up our property and factories. The point is that the growth in national and foreign debt implies that some economic pairs of opposites are moving further apart, and that spells eventual trouble. This is because in Nature, the pairs of opposites must complement each other in order to bring balance and harmony for organisms to survive and flourish.

American debt position is even worse in terms of foreign commerce. Since the beginning of the new millennium, we have needed to borrow over $2 billion per day from abroad to finance our trade deficit. This means that our foreign obligations have been rising at the rate of about $800 billion annually. Thus, in the first decade of the new millennium the foreign debt grew even faster than government debt, at a time when the living standard continued to fall. *Fig*. 5 displays the dramatic rise in our international borrowing since 2003, which includes the borrowing of private and public agencies. For instance, according to the Treasury Department, foreign investors hold over $1.4 trillion of Fannie Mae and Freddie Mac bonds. In a matter of four years from 2003 to 2007, we added over $6 trillion to our foreign debt.

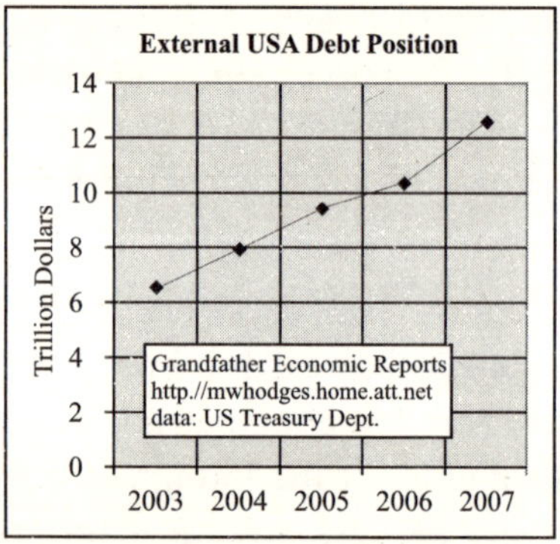

fig. 5: America's Foreign Debt
Source: mwhodges.home.att.net

The Negative Savings Rate

The period from 1950 to 1970 also preserved a rough balance between the real wage and productivity. *Figs*. 1 and 2 reveal that the production wage went up almost as fast as labour productivity at the time, but after 1973, the wage rate fell while productivity continued to increase. Productivity and wages are the two opposites in the labour market. Thus, the US labour market was in close balance until 1970, but an imbalance arose in the early 1970s and thereafter. Almost all economic theories agree that the real wage should rise with productivity; this is one case of rare consensus among economists. Fairness also demands that increased productivity should be rewarded with enhanced remuneration. At least the salary should not fall. But in the US, something happened after 1973 that had never occurred in its history before. The real wage actually fell while hourly output went up. So the labour-market imbalance is not only unprecedented, it is vast, and, as argued in Chapter 4, is the root cause of all other imbalances plaguing us today.

The negative to zero savings rate prevalent today is the direct result of the falling production wage. This is unprecedented and perhaps the biggest indicator of current economic imbalances. Take a look at *fig.* 6, which tracks the behaviour of our savings rate between 1949 and 2006. The graph shows that the savings rate went up from 1949 to 1974, then fell slightly, rose again, not surprisingly, in the recession of 1980 to 1982, but has steadily fallen ever since. In 2006 it was a negative 1.1 per cent. Imagine a nation with the highest per capita GDP in terms of purchasing power having a negative savings rate. No advanced economy can match our record today. Clearly, the savings rate rose in the 1950s and the 1960s, the decades when the production wage also jumped. This should not be a surprise. As your income rises, so does your ability to save. When the income falls, the savings rate automatically goes down.

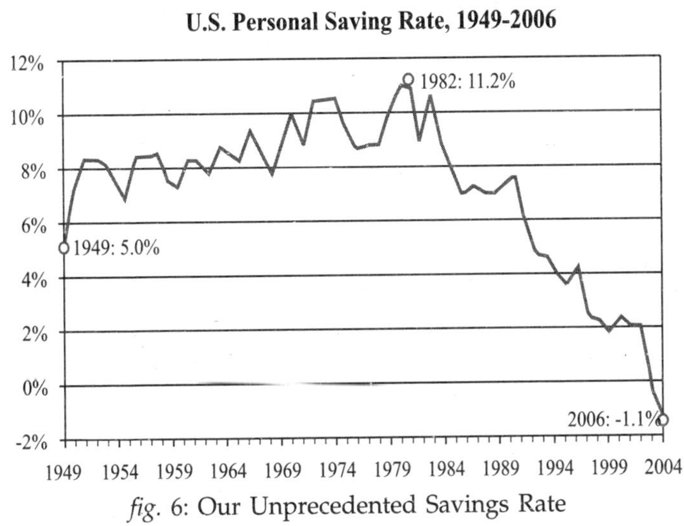

fig. 6: Our Unprecedented Savings Rate

Source: Inequality.org and The *ERP*, various issues.

There perhaps were other factors as well. Americans then did not rely much on government help and saving for a rainy day was an important practice. I recall the statement made by

President Kennedy in his inaugural address, "Ask not what your country can do for you — ask what you can do for your country."

You may have noticed that the savings rate fell after 1982 even though real family income went up, implying that the production wage is a better gauge of the living standard. This is because people should be able to save more when their living standard rises. The fact that family income rose does not mean that the living standard rose as well; in fact, the latter continued to fall, as indicated by sinking savings. During the late 1990s and 2000s the production wage actually rose slightly; then why did the savings rate not respond positively at that time? The reason is that the production wage fell faster than indicated by statistics, because the government changed the inflation-computing formula in 1996. Annual record from the *ERP* shows that the production wage was at $282 in 1980 and fell steadily to 258 by 1992, and then stayed at that level until 1995.

From 1996, when the inflation formula was changed, the production wage started to rise and reached a high of 282 in 2007. Thus, the new formula may have something to do with the rise in the wage in recent years. Even then the question remains: why was the savings rate negative in 2007 and fairly high in 1980 at 11 per cent, when the production wage was the same in both years. The answer may depend on the level of taxes paid by the middle class.

Since 1981, there has been a steady fall in the income tax rates imposed on individuals and corporations followed by a sharp rise in other levies such as the social security tax, Medicare tax, excise tax and the sales tax. For instance, the sales tax in most states today is about 7-8 per cent compared to less than 4 per cent in 1980. Similarly, the social security tax at 15.6 per cent is much higher than its 1980 level of 11 per cent. Since the income tax is progressive, that is, the rate rises with income, the burden of income taxes falls mostly on the wealthy and that of other levies mostly on the poor and the middle class. Thus, the tax burden of the well-to-do groups has declined sharply while that of the other groups has jumped. So the after-tax production wage, which does not apply to the wealthy has shrunk even faster than the pre-tax level since 1980.

The negative savings rates of 2000s are explained by the fact that the post-tax production wage is now much lower than that in 1980, even though the pre-tax levels are the same. The US savings behaviour today is so anomalous among advanced economies that it demands a sensible explanation, and I think the sharp decline in the post-tax production wage explains the unprecedented phenomenon adequately.

Consumer Debt

You may be wondering how there can be a negative savings rate. In other words, how can people spend more than they earn? Through borrowing! Just like our government, the American consumer has also been going into hock at record pace, especially since 2002. The overworked American has become an overborrowed American as well.

This is not surprising. It is the direct consequence of the declining pre and post-tax production wage. In order to maintain their lifestyle, people have been mortgaging their home equity and almost everything else. They don't own outright their furniture, cars, appliances, television and other big-ticket items. Their banks or credit-card companies partly own their possessions. *Fig.* 7 is very revealing. It shows that while household debt as a percentage of GDP has been steadily rising since 1957, the pace accelerated from 1981, when Reagan took over, and then again after 2001, when Bush II took over.

There must be something in their policies that sent our economy backwards in terms of national debt. We will study the details of their handiwork in Chapter 5. But it is more than a coincidence that President Bush adopts almost similar economic measures as President Reagan, and both times huge budget and trade gaps appear without bettering the lot of the average American. Both times the nation ends up borrowing a lot of money from abroad, while the savings rate falls and the production wage stagnates.

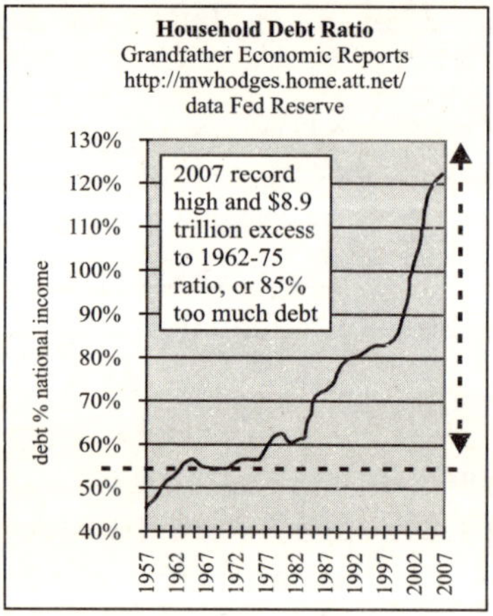

fig. 7: The Overborrowed American
Source: mwhodges.home.att.net

The Flourishing CEO

The fruit of productivity is production, which when sold is divided between the employer and the workers. From 1950 to 1970, both wages and hourly output went up; so both the producers and employees enjoyed higher living standards. The CEOs benefited, and so did their workers. But not after 1973, when the CEO incomes jumped while production workers suffered. This is because as productivity went up the production wage fell, so that CEO salaries grew even faster than productivity growth. The chairmen of the Fortune 100 minted money at the expense of their blue and white collar employees.

The managerial class had a reason to celebrate, but the working groups suffered. The earliest evidence available in this regard is from 1960. That year the average CEO wage, according to UFEnet.org, was 40 times the production wage;

by 2000 it had shot up to 525 times, and even in 2005, it was over 410 times. (See *Fig*. 6, which is provided by inequality.org from 1990 to 2005.) There is no reason to believe that the CEO income had jumped faster than the production wage prior to 1960. So from 1950 to 1970, income and wealth were properly distributed in the US, but by now a vast imbalance has appeared in this respect as well.

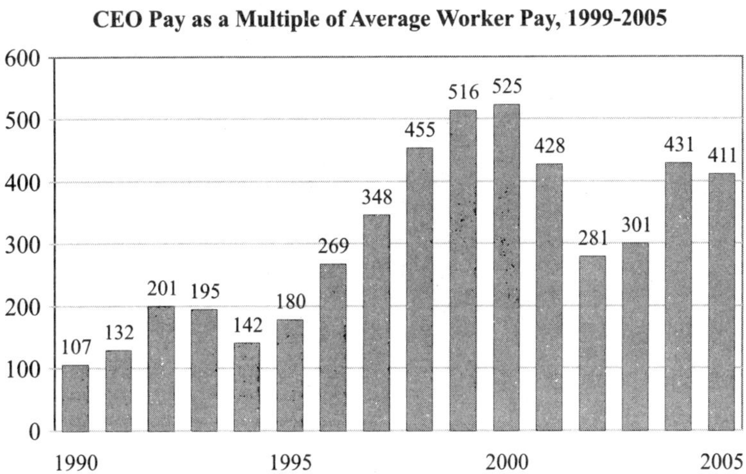

fig. 8: CEOs and Their Workers
Source: Inequality.org

The perception that there was a good balance between labour and management in capitalistic America was world over in the 1960s. It reminds me of the question posed by a reporter to India's Prime Minister Nehru visiting America in 1961: how can your socialistic policy be good for India? Nehru's response was immediate and precise, stating that he was trying to duplicate what American workers had achieved in getting a fair share of prosperity.

Going back to our earlier discussion, in terms of net worth, the richest 1 per cent of Americans held 125 times the median wealth in 1962; now they hold more than 190 times. See *fig*. 9.

Such wealth disparity is reminiscent of the 1920s, when mere 1 per cent of families owned over 36 per cent of total wealth, and we all know what happened in the next decade. Today, according to some studies, 1 per cent of American households own over 38 per cent of wealth, the worst in American **history**.[4]

Ratio of Top 1% Wealth to Median Wealth, 1962-2004

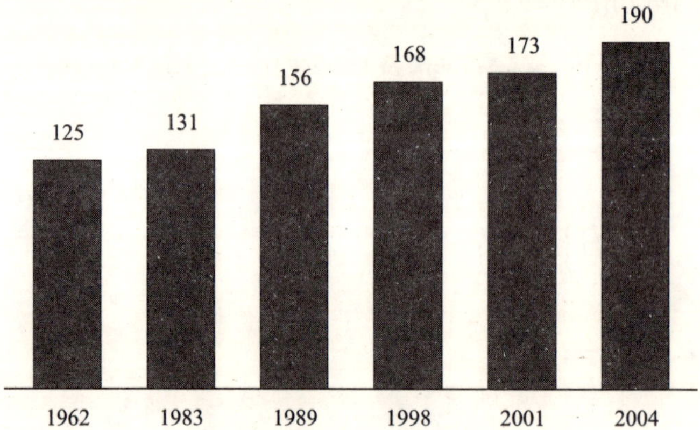

fig. 9: The US Distribution of Wealth

Source: Inequality.Org.

Wealth

MANUFACTURING AND SERVICES

Another area revealing a major imbalance today is in the relative strength of manufacturing versus services. With the erosion of our international competitiveness, manufacturing has declined sharply relative to the service sector. In 1960, nearly one in four workers was employed in manufacturing compared to less than 10 per cent in 2007 (*fig*. 10). You have to go as far back as 1830, when America was predominantly an agrarian economy, to see such a low level.

Why does manufacturing matter? There are two main reasons. First, manufacturing wage is substantially higher than the service wage, so that with the preponderance of service jobs, the average production wage must fall. Second, this development tends to create instability and imbalances in the economy, because it violates Markowitz's investment principle that no one should have most of his eggs in one basket. Markowitz argues that diversification is the best way to maximise return on one's investment. In the same way, production diversification among a number of sectors is the best way to maximise the nation's living standard. When a country produces few products, it does not have much to export. Today the US does not produce many goods it used to produce in the past. One by one, many industries such as television, VCRs, shoes, textiles have all but disappeared from the US soil. When the production base is narrow, export volume suffers and trade goes into deficit. Manufacturing loss is one reason why the US foreign trade shortfall has been soaring in recent years. Countries like Japan and China have much higher manufacturing production, and they are the current export powerhouses. When America was a major manufacturer, as from 1900 to 1970, it too had an export surplus. Those days are now a distant past.

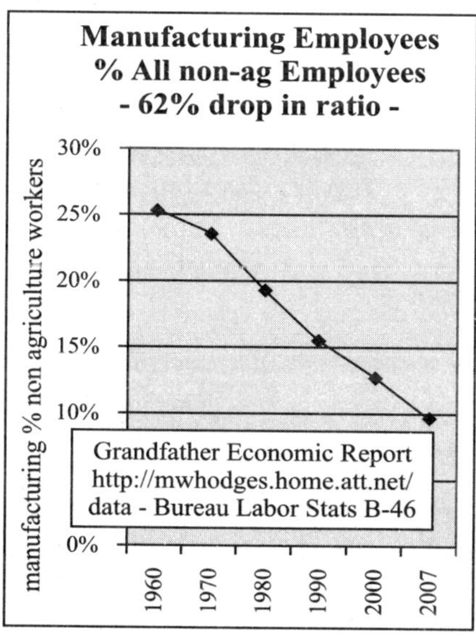

fig. 10: Manufacturing Job-Losses in the United States
Source: mwhodges.home.att.net

Conclusion

America has always been a land of liberty and prosperity. Today it is the land of liberty as well as vast financial imbalances. There is hardly any area in the economy that is not chafing under the burden of debt. Households, federal, state and local governments, small corporations and sole proprietorships are all in hock as never before, while the lenders belonging to the wealthy group of bigwig CEOs wallow in luxury. Oil profits have been soaring, even as the public faces mounting energy bills. The banking system is in a crisis mode, the housing market is crumbling, while the consumer is maxed out in credit cards. There are signs of stagflation similar to those in the 1970s. However, unlike today, in the 1970s wages were rising with inflation. The law of balancing the opposites says that when the two opposites are at war and don't even try reconciliation, moving away from each other and hitting their limits or boundaries, a great explosion may occur, leading to widespread destruction. Going back to the tornado analogy, when the opposites of extremely hot and cold airs have no path of slow diffusion but collide, they produce a massive whirlpool or cloud that can destroy everything in its path.

I am not sure we are there yet. But the rate at which our imbalances are piling up, the rate at which economic opposites are moving afar creating huge imbalances, I am certain that that pivotal point will arrive one day and possibly soon, unless we act in time to avoid economic convulsion.

The following provides a short list of the economic and political imbalanced pairs of opposites, some of which we have covered, while others will be covered later:

- Executive and legislative branches of government
- Government revenue and spending
- Corporate management and labour

- Consumer saving and spending
- Wages and purchasing power
- Export and import
- National debt and GDP
- Bubbles and their bursting (fear and greed)
- Inflation and interest rate
- Shortages and surpluses
- Consumption and pollution

We may be in a region where black swans appear frequently. These imbalances have occurred in spite of, or maybe because of, many advantages America has, such as the dollar being an international reserve currency and the US being a dominant world power. There are economists who believe that we have entered a period where the dollar is replaced by divergent currencies, including gold and other commodities.

A lot needs to be done including changing the value system; consumption is not a virtue, saving for a rainy day is. We may need continuous education at all levels, without compromising the individual freedom of choice. The government seems to be entangling itself with mortgage companies and banks, going away from the free enterprise economic system. I hope these actions are short-lived, limited, and only to correct the trajectory of the crisis. The CEOs need an alternate motivation other than just making money. There are plenty of examples recently, as with Enron or World Com, that show how easily corruption can spread.

Let us listen to our ancient wise men, introduce the balancing economic measures and reverse the trends that have brought us to the edge of a cliff. I will explore such measures in Chapter 6.

References

1. See Ravi Batra, The Myth of Free Trade, New York, Macmillan, 1993; and Common Sense Macroeconomics, Liberty Press, Dallas, 2004; Lester Thurow, The Future of Capitalism: How Today's Economic Forces Shape Tomorrow's World, New York: Morrow, 1996; Elizabeth Warren and Amelia Warren Tyagi,The Two Income Trap: Why Middle-class Mothers and Fathers Are Going Broke, New York: Basic Books, 2003;Lawrence Mishel and Jared Bernstein, The State of Working America, Washington D.C., Economic Policy Institute, 2003; Lou Dobbs, War on the Middle Class: How the Government, Big Business, and Special Interest Groups Are Waging War on the American Dream and How to Fight Back, New York: Viking Adult, 2006; Thom Hartmann, Screwed: The Undeclared War Against the Middle Class — And What We Can Do about It, San Francisco: Berrett-Koehler Publishers, 2007.
2. See dailykos.com
3. See Liz Pulliam Weston , "The Basics: What's a Homemaker Worth? The Shocking Truth," moneycentral.msn.com, 2008.
4. United for a Fair Economy, UFE: www.ufenet.org

3

Ideal Economy Concepts Since the Ancient Times

IT is commonly observed that in every creature, humans and animals alike, the urge for survival trumps every other urge. Life is dear to each and every one of us, and since economics deals primarily with producing the means of survival, the subject has been of interest to people since ancient times. "Men", said Karl Marx, "must be able to live in order to make history". Thus, the best way to create and distribute the means of livelihood has been explored by prominent scholars in virtually all civilisations.

We are facing tough economic problems today. Many questions pester us. How do we increase national output? How much should a worker be paid? How much revenue should the government collect from the public? Should the state own any property or engage in the production of goods? Every generation has to tackle such questions. Therefore, economics is an ancient subject, although modern economists prefer to date it back to Adam Smith, who wrote the *Wealth of Nations* in 1776.

According to written records, the earliest study of economics began in what is known as the Buddhist period, going as far back as the seventh century BCE. The period is named after the birth of the prophet Buddha in Nepal, the northern-most nation bordering India. Buddha was born as a prince, but left his family at the age of 29 to do hard penance in the Himalayan caves, and attained enlightenment ten years later. He preached his religion in India, and his disciples have left a rich record of contemporary and ensuing Indian society, along with its major kingdoms.

What is of great interest here is that, according to some Western historians, some kind of capitalism prevailed in north India during the Buddhist period; a few states were even organised as democracies, where kings were elected by the people.[1] Most American historians regard Athens as the birthplace of democracy. Buddhist literature shows that in this respect, India preceded Athens by at least two centuries. Athens' democracy appeared in the fifth century BCE, but India's arose in the seventh century BCE. This is also the period when metallic money came into vogue in India in the form of gold and silver coins, replacing the barter system that had hitherto facilitated the exchange of goods and services.

The discovery of money generated great prosperity. It enhanced trade among various kingdoms and gave rise to new industries, moneylending, urban centres and a whole range of new products that could be bought and sold in the market. Buddhist literature suggests that the state did not intervene in the economic activities of its subjects. Some moneylenders were fabulously wealthy, and some mercants were elected as kings. Ancient archives mention 16 major kingdoms, of which 8 were monarchies and the other 8 were republics, in which money played a big role at the time of elections. In other words, as in today's democracies, wealth dominated the politics of the Buddhist period in some states.

This was true not just in north India but also in south India. Some mercants were elected as kings and some as legislators. A few were Buddha's followers. Jataka, the main book of Buddhist writings, speaks of a few people of vast wealth, some of whom even had their own armies, and exerted great influence in the state. Wealth disparity was quite high among people, although there was no extreme poverty.

Buddhist literature only describes the state of the economy in India from the seventh to the fourth century BCE. It does not explain how the economy should be treated or administered in good and bad times. That task was performed later by a famous Indian philosopher named Vishnugupta, also known as Kautilya or Chanakya, who was a contemporary of Alexander the Great and appeared in the post-Buddha period, starting with the early fourth century BCE. Kautilya was actually a revolutionary, and lived in the kingdom of Magadha, with its capital at what is today known as Patna in the state of Bihar. Early on in his life he came into conflict with his king, named Dhanananda, who was greedy and tyrannical. The king's name literally translates as someone who finds joy in wealth, which indicates that the people of the republics as well as kingdoms were greatly interested in money. In fact, the contemporary Jataka literature gives us hints about high speculation, because it talks about rates of profit as high as 2000 per cent per year.

Kautilya may be regarded as the first economist in history. He was not only a great scholar, but also a rebel. Eventually he succeeded in overthrowing his king with the help of an army commander named Chandragupta Maurya, who then became the Magadhan emperor. Chandragupta appointed Kautilya as his prime minister, who faced the task of managing and reviving an economy that had been ruined because of anarchy and the previous king's greed and mismanagement. This is how Kautilya became an expert economist and went on to write a book called *Arthashastra*, which literally means *The Science of Wealth*. The title reminds us of Adam Smith's *Wealth of Nations*.

Kautilya's credentials as an economist are borne out by a clear understanding and analysis of the macro economy. The Mauryan Empire was vast and covered the entire portion of north India. Kautilya offers details about how to enrich the kingdom and raise the living standard of the masses, which is precisely what macroeconomics explores today. He argues in favour of a diversified economy that includes a wide variety of industries such as agriculture, mining and metals, fisheries, production of weapons, forestry, transportation and medicine. He also talks about the levels of wages and profits, both of which should be reasonable to generate prosperity. In his view, excessive profits generate inflation because they can exist only if prices far exceed costs. So inflation can be avoided if prices are reasonable. Such advice is particularly needed in today's oil industry, where prices are sharply above the cost of production, and profits have skyrocketed. Kautilya also suggests that a good economy requires good wages; otherwise, workers will suffer, shirk work and be unproductive. Above all, a prosperous economy needs a virtuous king or the head of the state. Some interesting excerpts from *Arthashastra* are as follows:

> In the happiness of his subjects lies the king's happiness, in their welfare his welfare. He shall not consider as good only that which pleases him but treat as beneficial to him whatever pleases his subjects. . . .
>
> Hence the king shall be ever active in the management of the economy. The root of wealth is (productive) activity and lack of it creates material distress. In the absence of (such) activity, both current prosperity and future growth will be destroyed. A king can achieve the desired objectives and an abundance of riches by undertaking economic activity.

These ideas are similar to what policymakers believe in various democracies today. Kautilya advises his king to look after the welfare of his people "by undertaking economic activity", which includes the building of roads, waterways, irrigation facilities, settlement of immigrants, forestry, weapons of war — especially elephants — and provision of tax incentives to increase worker productivity. Elsewhere, Kautilya writes that an illustrious king is one who "endears himself to his people by enriching them and doing good to them. Such a disciplined king should keep away from another's wife and not covet another's property".

It is clear that Kautilya's ideal ruler excludes Bill Clinton, who while in office often found it difficult to keep away from married and unmarried women. The heads of state in the US, Europe, Canada, Australia and India — presidents and prime ministers — recognise today that they will not be re-elected if the economy is in bad shape. If unemployment is high, prices are rising fast or real wages are falling, the incumbents are usually defeated by challengers. So in their self-interest, the government officials seek to generate a strong and efficient economy with high employment, stable prices and growing prosperity. They increase government spending or cut taxes and interest rates to fight joblessness; they reduce the supply of money to fight inflation. Kautilya wants to achieve the same goals for his people, but he goes a step further. He exhorts his king to be virtuous not because of self-interest to stay in office but for the sake of people's welfare. So Kautilya was the first scholar in history who not only analysed the importance of various industries to generate prosperity, but also explored the requirements of an ideal economy. He realised that an ideal economy could not exist without an ideal king: "If the king is energetic, his subjects will be equally energetic. If he is slack and lazy in performing his duties, the subjects will also be lax and thereby eat into his wealth."

According to Kautilya, a virtuous king — the president or prime minister in today's world — is one who does not covet another's wife or property and keep his senses under control, is ever active in promoting the security and welfare of the people, appoints wise and intelligent people as his officers, who are not afraid to remind him of his duties and, if necessary, reprimand him for his bad conduct. In other words, a good king does not surround himself with yes-men:

> A Raja-rishi (great king) shall always respect those counselors and *purohitas* (advisers) who warn him of the dangers of transgressing the limits of good conduct, reminding him sharply of the times prescribed for various duties and caution him even when he errs in private.

Kautilya also believes in private property and favours balancing the government budget without excessive taxation:

> A king with depleted treasury will eat into the very vitality of both citizens and country people. Either on the occasion of opening new settlements or on any other emergent occasions, remission of taxes shall be made.

In other words, the king should raise adequate revenue to avoid a depleted treasury. This is a call for balancing the budget. In fact, *Arthashastra* has a long chapter describing the duties and responsibilities of the collector-general of taxes and fines; how government accounts are to be maintained and so on.

However, in emergencies such as famines, there should be tax remission. Today, we call it fiscal policy to fight a recession. Thus, Kautilya is not an advocate of big government, nor of budget deficits. He believes that the king should enrich his people; this means that taxes cannot be exorbitant; yet they cannot be so low that the treasury is depleted and the king cannot carry on the indispensable work of security and maintaining law and order. The king may also engage in retailing, i.e. buy and sell local and imported goods to earn a profit, so that taxes remain low.

Kautilya also favours some type of social welfare for those who are handicapped and cannot support themselves. He writes:

> The king shall provide the orphans, the aged, the infirm, the afflicted, and the helpless with maintenance. He shall also provide subsistence to helpless women when they are carrying and also to the children they give birth to.

Kautilya seeks to reward honest and productive taxpayers with tax incentives and punish those who shirk work. He says:

> Lands prepared for cultivation shall be given to taxpayers for life. Unprepared lands shall not be taken away from those who are preparing them for cultivation. Lands may be confiscated from those who do not cultivate them and given to others; if cultivators pay their taxes easily, they may be favourably supplied with grains, cattle, and money.

Kautilya even believes in profit sharing:

> Whoever stays away from any kind of cooperative construction shall send his servants and bullocks to carry on his work, shall have a share in the expenditure, but shall have no claim to the profit.

Here there are two important ideas. First, a person can be involved in a project by utilising his servants and bullocks, and for this he will receive due compensation from the expenditure; but he will have no claim to the profit. Second, the profit will be distributed among those who directly work on the project. Direct work thus, is more important than absentee work.

A section of *Arthashastra* deals with forcign trade. Kautilya writes that goods may be imported by mercants or by the government, and then sold at a reasonable price. He writes:

> That merchandise of the king which is of local manufacture shall be centralised; imported merchandise shall be distributed in several markets for sale. Both kinds of merchandise shall be favourably sold to the people. He shall avoid such large profits as will harm the people.

Thus, Kautilya argues again and again that profit should be reasonable and not so high as to harm the people through exorbitant prices. Kautilya also believes in export incentives through tax remission to exporters.

No work on macroeconomics can be complete without a chapter on money and its value. Kautilya does not disappoint us in this regard. He is very concerned about the quality of metallic money and offers a complete chapter on how coins are to be manufactured, regulated and standardised. Thus he writes:

> The State Goldsmith shall employ artisans to manufacture gold and silver coins from the bullion of citizens and country people.
>
> When the quality of a coin . . . is lowered, the artisans shall be penalised mildly. When its weight is less than the standard weight, they shall be punished harder. Deception in balance or weights shall be punished with the highest punishment. Deception in the exchange of manufactured coins shall also be punished with the highest punishment.
>
> Whoever causes gold or silver articles to be manufactured in any place other than the mint or without being noticed by the state goldsmith shall be fined 12 *pans*, while the artisan who does that work shall, if found out, be punished with twice the above fine.
>
> The examiner of coins shall regulate currency both as a medium of exchange and as legal tender admissible into the treasury.

Thus, Kautilya is worried about the debasement of money. He is aware of its importance as a medium of exchange, prescribes standards for the manufacture of coins, makes sure that their supply is kept under control and provides penalties for those engaged in the counterfeit of money.

Another chapter in *Arthashastra* deals with the textile industry especially with the department of weaving. Here we get hints about Kautilya's attitude toward wages and female labour, because the textile industry was dominated by women workers. Kautilya writes:

> The Superintendent of Weaving shall employ qualified persons to manufacture threads, coats, cloths, and ropes.
>
> Wages shall be fixed accordingly as the threads spun are fine, coarse or of middle quality and in proportion to a greater or less quantity manufactured, and in consideration of the quantity of thread spun, those shall be presented with oil and dried cakes of *myrobalan* fruits. They may also be made to work on holidays by payment of special rewards.
>
> Wages shall be cut short, if making allowance for the quality of raw material, the quantity of the threads spun out is found to fall short.
>
> Weaving may also be done by those artisans who are qualified to turn out a given amount of work in a given time and for a fixed amount of wages. Those women who can present themselves at the weaving house shall at dawn be enabled to exchange their spinning for wages. If the superintendent looks at the face of such women or talks about any other work, he shall be punished with the first amercement (fine). Delay in paying the wages shall be punished with the middlemost amercement.

Two ideas stand out from these paragraphs. First, Kautilya does not condone discrimination on grounds of sex; sexual harassment by male superintendents is to be punished by fines. Second, he believes in setting wages consistent with worker productivity. Thus, high quality work is to be rewarded with higher wages and low quality work with lower compensation.[2]

In short, Kautilya stands out as the first economist in history. He is brilliant and thorough in his examination of the macro economy. His views display compassion and common sense, and are designed to enrich the citizenry. Much like macroeconomics today, he opts for a mixed economy, where private enterprise is complemented by a wide variety of government activities such as internal and external security, printing of money, construction of roads and highways, bridges, ports, airports, firefighting, health care and welfare for the handicapped. Kautilya penalises sexual harassment and discrimination, offers wages matching productivity, and makes sure that profits are reasonable so that prices stay low. Furthermore, unlike the governments today he wants to balance the treasury's budget to avoid building up debt, and control the supply of money to avoid its debasement. His compassion is matched by practicality and his system of rewards and fines displays a keen understanding of human nature.

Some provisions from *Arthashastra*, or the *Science of Wealth*, can constitute a stellar guide in creating an ideal economy today. This is because the Mauryan Empire became very wealthy after Kautilya took charge. Chandragupta's grandson Ashoka is known as Ashoka the Great. He took *Arthashastra* to heart, became a truly virtuous king, created a vast Indian empire that stretched from Afghanistan all the way to Burma, and greatly enriched his people.

Kautilya's work exerted vast influence on Indian economic thought for centuries, because India remained wealthy for a long time. For ages, the nation was known as a golden sparrow. Even Columbus was fascinated with tales of India's fabulous wealth, and when he left town to circle the globe, his objective was to find a western route to the opulent land. In fact, when his ship came ashore, he thought he had succeeded in his mission, but he had actually discovered America and called the natives Indians. However ancient India, which was ruined by anarchy and ceaseless warfare among states in the Buddhist period, could not have prospered without Kautilya's brilliant work and understanding of the functioning of the macro economy.

Plato and Aristotle

To my mind, Kautilya was the first economist in history; but he was not the first to offer economic ideas. There were others before him, notably Plato and Aristotle, who had also delved in the subject, but they fell way short of Kautilya's thoroughness and brilliance. Plato offers a rudimentary discussion of demand and supply. He writes: "They exchange with one another, and one gives and another receives under the idea that the exchange will be for their good."[3] Apparently this idea refers to demand and supply for goods. The source of demand, in Plato's view, are people's primary wants, which are food, clothing and shelter. These wants give rise to various occupations including husbandmen, weavers, home builders, shoemakers, carpenters and blacksmiths. Exchange among the workers creates the need for mercants, who stock goods made at home and abroad. This need for mutual exchange gives rise to the establishment of a state, which is thus an expression of people's wants. But Plato's individual is subordinate to the state, although the author does exhort the government to take care of the handicapped and those crippled in war.

Plato's ideal state comprises 5,040 people and he believes in population control; if the population falls below this number, people should be given incentives to procreate; and if the number is exceeded, then some people should be sent into the colonies. Thus, the state has a large role in regulating people's lives. Similarly, Plato does not believe in market-determined prices, even though he lucidly described the practice of exchange. He opts for regulated prices. Not surprisingly, he does not like the institution of private property, either, favouring community property instead.

Aristotle differs from Plato in many ways. Aristotle's state arises from the fact that "man is naturally a social animal", and likes to live in company.[4] There is no economic motive that creates the state. Aristotle also dislikes Plato's communism wherein people share their property with each other, including their wives and children so as to avoid jealousies and quarrels. To Aristotle, individuals have some rights of their own and they also have duties. His biggest contribution lies in making a distinction between value in use and value in exchange, an idea that is till accepted by economists today. A commodity may be useful but it may have small value in terms of monetary exchange, because there it depends on the market price. Money to Aristotle is something coveted by all because of its ability to satisfy our needs, but he insists that its acquisition is not an end in itself. He concedes that people are naturally acquisitive but he does not condone the practice. This should not be happening in a good society. This is the closest that Aristotle comes as far as an ideal economy is concerned. But his economy is part of the social order and not something that needs to be improved upon in itself.

However, Aristotle does believe in the idea of balance. He suggests that people should not be overly acquisitive, nor should they be poor. There should be a happy middle ground in their lives.

The Rise of Capitalism

Apart from Kautilya and the Greek thinkers, there is very little discussion of economic ideas among scholars until the rise of Western-style capitalism in the seventeenth century. In the thirteenth century, the Christian scholar Thomas Aquinas did explore the notions of regulated prices and interest rates, suggesting that both of them should be controlled to make goods and lending affordable to the public. There is a just price and a just interest rate in his view. But how the economy works or markets function, are not discussed by him.

The earliest economic theory dealing with European capitalism is known as mercantilism; the idea developed primarily in England in the 1620s and then spread to the rest of Europe. The theory argues that a nation's prosperity depends upon its horde of bullion — gold and silver. So the state should try to acquire bullion by exporting as many goods as possible and by limiting imports through protectionist measures.

Mercantilism also advocates extensive state control of the economy. It encourages the formation of monopolies for profit, especially those held by the state. It holds that a tightly regulated economy generates prosperity. This thought was very popular in Europe in the seventeenth and eighteenth centuries. But internationally it created numerous wars, as governments tried to corner the markets in their colonies and discourage imports from other nations. In the end, bloody warfare and the system's inherent contradictions that generated poverty led to its demise.

Adam Smith

After Kautilya, it is not until Adam Smith that we see a systematic and thorough attempt to explain the functioning of an economy. Smith's *Wealth of Nations* is today regarded as a masterpiece, but many of its integral ideas can be found in *Arthashastra*. Kautilya advances the notion that economic prosperity depends on a diversified system with a large number of industries. So does Smith. Kautilya argues that the state has a strong role to play in people's economic development by providing infrastructure, justice and defence against foreign enemies. Smith does the same. Kautilya suggests that the poor should not be taxed, and the government should balance its budget. Smith too says so. Kautilya argues in favour of stable and sound money that prevents rising prices and hence exorbitant profits. Smith also sees the need for profit moderation, but through the means of strong competition among businessmen. Kautilya makes sure that wages are consistent with people's productivity, whereas Smith argues that competition among firms and workers leads to the same outcome. Even regarding foreign trade, their views are similar. They both like to impose tariffs if the foreign nation does the same.

Of course, there are differences between the two writers, and that is to be expected in works that are separated by centuries and stand apart geographically. *Arthashastra*'s state or king plays a much larger role in the enrichment of people, whereas Smith would have minimal official intervention in the economy. Kautilya also derides intervention, but he wants to make sure that no one starves in the kingdom, or that the needy are cared for. He wants the king to undertake some economic activity and earn income so as to limit the level of taxation. Thus, if Smith is the precursor of modern economics, Kautilya is the precursor of ideas that generate today's mixed economies, in which the government is expected to solve people's economic problems in an essentially private enterprise system. In this respect, modern nations are closer to Kautilya's conception of the state than Smith's.

However, Smith makes a towering contribution in terms of economic logic. What is an ideal economy? The one that, according to Smith, has sufficient competition among firms in every industry. Competition among businesses, consumers and workers generates prosperity and material happiness. Scholars such as Aquinas had denounced people's greed and penchant for money as creators of anarchy. Smith argued to the contrary, saying that greed and self-interest generate a rich society, as long as there is competition among people.

Smith observed that when a person starts a business he wants to make money, and if he has to compete with other firms, his self-interest will goad him to produce a high quality product at the cheapest possible price. Otherwise, he will not be able to sell his goods. Workers, on the other hand, have to work hard in order to get promotion and high salary, when they compete with each other. Their self-interest makes them highly productive, which in turn will lower production cost for their employer, who is then able to charge a lower price. Finally, consumers in their self-interest go to that seller who offers a good product at the lowest price. This way, everyone's self-interest ensures that high quality goods are produced by qualified workers at the lowest price. So greed is not bad as long as the state does not intervene to pass laws that hinder competition among firms and workers. Self-interest is thus Adam Smith's famous "invisible hand" that brings producers, employees and consumers together to generate a productive economy and a high living standard. This way, the celebrated author denounced the state monopolies and labourer's guilds that restrained completion among workers.

Is the state totally unnecessary for prosperity? No, said Smith, but the government should limit its activities to justice, defence against foreign enemies, and the provision of infrastructure. He writes:

> According to the system of natural liberty, the sovereign has only three duties to attend to; three duties of great importance, indeed, but plain and intelligible to common understanding: first, the duty of protecting the society from the violence and invasion of other independent societies; secondly, the duty of protecting, as far as possible, every member of society from the injustice or oppression of every other member of it, or the duty of establishing an exact administration of justice; and, thirdly, the duty of erecting and maintaining certain public works and certain public institutions, which it can never be for the interest of any individual, or small number of individuals, to erect and maintain; because the profit could never repay the expense to any individual or small number of individuals, though it may frequently do much more than repay it to a great society.[5]

This is Kautilya talking in Smith's guise. He offers similar words — the king should be virtuous and treat his people with equality and kindness, maintain a large and powerful army to defeat foreign enemies, and build public works such as roads, waterways, forests, ports and so on to enrich his people.

Classical Economics

Smith founded a school of thought that today is known as classical economics, for which there were some other contributors as well. The most well known among them was a French writer named Jean Baptiste Say. Smith dealt with productive efficiency and the functioning of markets in terms of a *laissèz faire* policy, where the government does not intervene. Say argued that such a system provides a quality job to everyone seeking it, that is to say, it is prone to creating full employment.

Say's argument proceeds by way of his well-known dictum — namely, supply creates its own demand. The idea is that the supply of goods and services in a nation automatically equals their demand, so that whatever a firm produces finds customers and there is no overproduction. The notion of overproduction is very important to maintain full employment, because if goods are not sold then the employer has to lay off workers.

Although Say offered his analysis in terms of a barter economy where goods exchange for other goods without the presence of money, other writers such as Alfred Marshall and A.C. Pigou developed the argument in a monetary economy, reaching the same conclusion that a free market system automatically generates full employment without the help of the government. In fact, they went further by saying that government intervention in the form of minimum legislation or labour union laws may actually cause unemployment. So they were adamantly opposed to any kind of government regulation of the economy.

However, there were frequent recessions and periods of high joblessness during the nineteenth century. At that time, the classical economists would say, "Give the system time to heal itself." They argued that recessions are temporary in a *laisséz faire* system, unlikely to last longer than two years. Their theory ruled out depressions, which in any case could be blamed on government intervention.

Classical economists believed in small government with balanced budgets and low taxation. They also opposed raising money supply to fight unemployment, because that would only be inflationary. In short, classical policy called for the government to keep its hands off the economy in good and bad times.

Karl Marx

The free market system that the classicists championed seemed to have a number of flaws. It suffered from occasional recessions and periods of high unemployment. People's wages were also low and not commensurate with their productivity, while profits tended to be high. So the system's theory did not match its performance. It had its critics and the most influential among them was Karl Marx, who offered a new type of economic model to explain the misery of the poor. In his view, "The history of all existing society is the history of class struggle".[6] While this is an extremely narrow view of history, there is a germ of truth in it.

According to Marx, every society has two main classes — those who own property and those who do not — the proprietor class and the rest. The proprietors own the means of production, and the livelihood of others depends on the sweet will of the former. Under capitalism, for instance, capitalists or the bourgeoisie own factories and others offer their labour for wages, which are rarely above subsistence. Extremely low wages in turn, generate extraordinary profits. This is what creates conflict between the two classes, i.e. between the capitalists and the proletariat. Thus, high profits of proprietors coupled with low wages of workers generate the class struggle under capitalism. This is the main and inevitable source of social conflict.

Marx sought to prove that labour was exploited under all forms of capitalism — competitive as well as monopolistic. He did this by asserting that labour is the only source of production. Capital and natural resources are also necessary for production, but all machinery and raw materials were produced by labour in the past. Thus, in the end, labour, current and past, is the only factor responsible for production. With labour being the only productive factor, all profits are unfair, which means that capitalism is nothing but an exploitation of the labouring class. Thus, to Marx all profits are undeserved.

How does the bourgeoisie ensure a persistently low wage, when wages depend upon the demand and supply of labour? The answer is: by means of labour-saving technology. Marx argues that whenever labour becomes scarce and threatens to raise wages sharply, the capitalist introduces labour-saving inventions to reduce demand for labour and hence the wage rate. Employing this method, salaries rarely rise above subsistence.

Besides profit, the capitalist is also interested in an exalted social status that depends on the size of his wealth. So he must save money to accumulate wealth and thus enhance his standing. Excessive saving, however, leads to a fall in national demand as well as a decline in the rate of profit, which is really the return on capital. This fall in demand leads to recessions and depressions.

During these downturns, the rich capitalists gobble up smallish firms, so that competition declines. In fact, Marx predicted that Europe's corporations would increasingly become oligopolies and even monopolies over time, and wages would fall even more. Eventually, a mega depression would come and the impoverished proletariat would overthrow the capitalist class in a revolution. The workers would then start a new phase in history, where the means of production would be owned collectively and class conflict would disappear. As private property ceases, there would be no class divisions, resulting in economic communism of the kind first envisioned by Plato. People would then share their property; there would be no more inequality in society and an ideal economy would be born, where everyone would be peaceful and prosperous.

Such then is the Marxist version of an ideal economy — complete economic equality, with no conflict whatsoever, and no state either. Why would you need a government when people have no more quarrels?

Needless to say, Marxism has not lived up to its claims. Some of its forecasts have indeed come true; capitalism is no longer competitive; mega corporations abound all over the world. Such forecasts have been accurate, but Marx's major predictions of an impoverished working class in Europe, a proletariat revolution and the birth of communism are nowhere in sight. Furthermore, communism does not seem to be possible or even desirable. How can inequality vanish altogether when people are born with innate differences in physical and intellectual ability? Furthermore, the absence of any diversity can make life very boring. Marxist contradictions are obvious and too many, and we need not spend a lot of space highlighting them. It is clear that the Marxist ideal is no ideal at all.

Keynesian Economics

Marx did offer a penetrating insight in the working of capitalism, namely the role of low consumer demand in the creation of recessions and depressions. But because of his extreme hostility to capitalism, this insight went unnoticed by the economic profession, which continued to side with Say's dictum that supply creates its own demand, so that long-term overproduction and hence depressions are impossible in a private enterprise system. Thus, classical economics remained the accepted doctrine for more than a century. It was demolished during the 1930s and the Great Depression, when unemployment soared to record heights, and remained high for the entire decade. Classical claims of a shallow and temporary recession in a self-healing system then appeared hollow. Established economists were forced by facts to admit that the system did not automatically generate full employment.

It was in this background that a British economist, John Maynard Keynes, wrote his *General Theory* and offered the first coherent critique of Say's law of markets. Keynes debunked the idea that supply creates its own demand, because people save money from their incomes causing reduction in their spending and demand. The classical economists had handled the effect of savings by suggesting that while people save money, businesses invest money by buying machinery or building factories and if the investment spending offsets the level of savings, supply is still equal to demand, leaving no overproduction behind.

The idea of overproduction is at the heart of macroeconomics, because overproduction leads to recessions, layoffs and hence unemployment. Classical economists went to great length to show that national supply cannot exceed national demand for long, because anytime this happens, the interest rate falls, inducing companies to borrow more money from banks and spending it to expand their business; consumers, on the other hand, are moved to cut their savings and thus raise their spending. This process continues until spending by consumers and companies rises to the level of supply. This way, any overproduction or recession that may occur because of excessive savings vanishes in a matter of one or two years, thereby eliminating unemployment swiftly. This is how the classicists ruled out depressions and even long recessions.

But the Great Depression defied the classical logic. Overproduction and hence unemployment went on and on; economists around the globe were uneasy about the defiant production systems but no one could explain why Say's law had a faulty logic. It was left to Keynes to demolish and bury this law. He started with a simple observation that the interest rate does not have a strong impact on consumer spending and hence savings. Rather, people's incomes determine their saving and spending behaviour. Consequently, when the interest rate declines, consumer spending may not rise at all, or may rise only sluggishly in a recession where incomes fall; similarly, business investment also may not rise, when goods are piling up on shelves. In these circumstances, savings may exceed investment for a long time, leading to general overproduction and long-term unemployment.

Keynes suggested that this is what had happened at the start of 1929, when the stock market crashed, depressing spending from consumers as well as producers. Such decline in demand had left the factories idle. Keynes then went on to recommend an anti-*laisséz faire* policy. He suggested that since the public was averse to increasing spending in the 1930s, the government should borrow money from the treasury, spend it on public works projects, and thus jump-start the economy. In other words, the government should have a massive budget deficit, over and above it already had in a faltering economy.

To the orthodox economist, trained in the classical logic, this was blasphemy. The general thinking was that the government should not intervene, because its intervention makes matters worse. So Keynes' recommendation went nowhere, and the depression continued unabated. As late as 1939, the unemployment rate in the US was 18 per cent. That was the year Second World War started. Germany, France and Britain were engulfed in a bloody war that required massive spending on weapons. No economist could object to the huge budget deficits that now ensued. America also had to raise its spending sharply to aid its allies. Within a few years, unemployment disappeared, and the public saw the wisdom of Keynes' ideas in times of a depression. That is when Keynesian economics began to replace the classical thought.

Monetarism

Keynes had undertaken a total demolition of classical views. He had offered new theories of consumption and savings, the rate of interest, bond and stock markets, labour market and so on. Above all, he had solved the depression dilemma. He became the most celebrated economist in the world, but died soon after the war.

Following Keynes' death, his theories fell into the hands of those who lacked his breadth and vision. Keynes had actually offered two types of policies — one to fight a depression, and another to fight a recession. Depression could be defeated only through massive budget deficits, but a recession could be fought with a small budget deficit along with a slight increase in money supply to bring down the interest rate. The first was the policy of fiscal expansion, the second the policy of monetary expansion. He also suggested that fiscal deficits should be followed by fiscal surpluses, so that the government budget would be balanced over the course of the business cycle. His followers, however, thought that monetary and fiscal policies could be used to permanently reduce unemployment, and banish recessions and poverty forever. They came up with a bankrupt idea called deficit financing.

Keynes had argued that high income inequality under capitalism creates a glut of savings and thus an occasional shortfall in national demand, leading to periodic unemployment. The neo-Keynesians argued that this tendency of capitalism could be neutralised if the government ran annual budget deficits and financed them by printing money. This way, extra government spending would add to the low private spending and thus keep demand and hence employment high. The followers of Keynes thus ignored his recommendation to balance the budget over the business cycle; instead, they sought to defeat the cycle itself by means of yearly monetary expansion. They, of course, knew this could result in inflation, but to them, slight inflation was a better evil than the curse of periodic unemployment.

The idea of deficit financing had its critics, notably Milton Friedman, who warned that monetary expansion could get out of hand and generate intolerable inflation, but the neo-Keynesians were in charge of government policy, especially under President Kennedy, and they persisted with their idea. By the end of the 1960s, inflation indeed began to multiply, but the neo-Keynesians were not deterred by it. By the end of the 1970s, however, inflation was rising at the rate of 1 per cent a month, and now even they conceded defeat. This is how Friedman's brand of economics, called monetarism, gained prominence.

Friedman sought to replace Keynesian thought altogether, and revive the classical orthodoxy. He suggested that money supply, not investment, was the primary variable in moving the economy. Keynes had focused on the lack of investment relative to savings as the main cause of recessions and depressions, whereas Friedman argued that it was the sudden fall in the supply of money from banks that usually preceded recessions. Friedman's economic policy thus focused on *laisséz faire* along with a policy of monetary stability. Money supply, according to Friedman, should be allowed to rise at the rate of long-term GDP growth, which approximates 4 per cent per year. This would keep prices stable and also avoid recessions.

This was a sharp departure from the neo-Keynesian view that had condoned money growth as high as 10 per cent per year during the 1970s. In the late 1970s and the early 1980s, when inflationary expectations had captured the public, monetarism offered the best solution and was practised by then Fed Chairman, Paul Volcker. This way inflation was tamed, and Keynesian economics discredited.

Supply-side Economics

In 1980, the world economy was on a perilous course. Governments had enacted huge budget deficits and deficit financing for many years and were then paying a big price for it in terms of high inflation and job losses. A new brand of economics now appeared to fill the vacuum of ideas. Monetarism was popular on the money side, but on the fiscal side, an economist named Arthur Laffer argued for massive cuts in income tax rates to stimulate the economy and get rid of high inflation and unemployment at the same time. He called his measure the supply-side economics. The Republican presidential candidate, Ronald Reagan, seized this idea and campaigned on the issue against the unpopular incumbent, Jimmy Carter. Reagan won handsomely and later sought the help of his economic adviser, Alan Greenspan, to convince Congress to legislate the tax cut.

Greenspan had frequently opposed this idea during the 1970s for fear that it would exacerbate the federal deficit and ignite inflation. But he flip-flopped in 1981 and offered his support to the tax-cut legislation, which was passed in June. Greenspan argued that the income tax cut would stimulate so much saving and investment that the resulting high GDP growth would actually raise the tax revenue substantially while reducing inflation and unemployment at the same time. This, combined with spending reduction, would also lower the budget deficit. To most economists, the whole idea appeared as voodoo economics, something too good to be true. How the tax cut could possibly lower the budget deficit was beyond their comprehension, especially when the spending cuts had never been enacted in the past and were unlikely in the future.

The sceptics turned out to be right. Government spending remained on the same trajectory as before and the tax cut reduced the revenue so much that by 1982, the federal deficit more than doubled. As government borrowing shot up, even as Volcker followed monetarism to curb inflation, interest rates soared, creating the worst recession since the Great Depression. Greenspan then made another flip-flop and advised Congress to raise not the income tax but several excise taxes to generate more revenue. But the deficit kept rising. So in 1983, the government sharply raised the social security tax and the self-employment tax. Income tax is borne mostly by the wealthy, whereas other taxes burden mostly the low-income groups. This way, from 1981 to 1983, the tax burden was transformed massively from the rich to the poor and the middle class. This transformation was unprecedented, causing the distortion in the character of the economy.

Suppose you lower the rich man's tax by $100 and raise the poor man's tax by the same amount. Consumer spending will then fall by close to $100. This is because the poor will have to cut their spending by the amount of the tax rise, while the rich, with needs already satisfied, will mostly save their tax reduction. As spending declines, overproduction will occur and discourage investment. So the supply-side policy cannot possibly produce the results it promises. You cannot defy the laws of addition and subtraction. Other things remaining the same, GDP growth then has to fall. This is precisely what happened. From 1950 to 1980, the US economy grew annually at the rate of 3.9 per cent, but because of the tax transformation, growth fell to 2.8 per cent in the 1980s, rose slightly to 3 per cent in the 1990s, and then fell again to 2.7 per cent in the 2000s.[7] The blight of the supply-side economics continues with no end in sight. The moral is that you cannot pass the tax burden onto the backs of the poor and expect a healthy economy.

Conclusion

By now, I have given you a brief description of how economic thought has evolved through the ages, from ancient times till today. Every generation has some version of what an ideal economy and society should be. Kautilya's ideal could be produced only by a virtuous government in a mixed economy, where private enterprise is complimented by a benevolent government activity that cares for the handicapped. Plato believed in communism, as did Marx, where property is shared. Aristotle's ideal permits some degree of private ownership along with low income and wealth disparity. Thomas Aquinas favoured official controls over prices and interest rates to keep profits reasonable and necessitates affordable to the public. Mercantilists believed in a powerful state and restrained competition to generate high trade surplus for the nation, an idea that was later denounced by Adam Smith and other classical economists such as J.B. Say. The classicists argued that high competition alone generates an efficient economy with full employment and high living standards for all. Keynes, by contrast, sought to inject the helping hand of the government in the otherwise classical world. Friedman opted for a sound money policy to create a good economy. Finally, the supply-siders such as Greenspan seek to offer tax incentives to the wealthy to encourage savings, investment and growth. It is the supply-side economics that now reigns the realm of macroeconomics. It is found in modern macro texts and, of course, in government policy. Whatever imbalances appear in the world today are attributable primarily to the supply-side school.

Endnotes

1. See, for instance, E.W. Hopkins, "The Period of Sutras, Epics and Law-Books", in *The Cambridge History of India*, vol. I, ed. E. J. Rapson, London: Cambridge University Press, 1935; C.A.F. Rhys-Davids, "Economic Conditions according to Early Buddhist Literature", in *The Cambridge History of India*, vol. I; Max Weber, *The Religion of India*, Glencoe, The Free Press, 1958; H.G. Rawlinson, *India: A Short Cultural History*, New York: Fredrick Praeger, 1952.
2. Excerpts from *Arthashastra* have been taken from two sources — *Kautilya. Arthashastra*, tr. R. Shamasastry, Bangalore: Government Press, 1915, pp. 51-185; and Wikipedia, *Arthashastra Encyclopedia*.
3. Quoted from L.H. Haney, *History of Economic Thought*, New York: Macmillan, 1936, p. 57.
4. Ibid.
5. Adam Smith, *An Inquiry into the Nature and Causes of the Wealth of Nations*, Indianapolis, Ind.: Liberty Press, 1976, pp. 687-88.
6. Karl Marx and F. Engels, "The Communist Manifesto", in *Essential Works of Marxism*, ed. A. P. Mendel, New York: Bantam, 1965, p. 13.
7. See the *ERP*, 2008 and other years.

4

The Wage Gap
A Unified Theory of Macroeconomics

THE week of 19 September 2008 was apparently a turning point for the US, moving us away from dominance in matters of the world economy and politics. Wall Street would never be the same again. Within a span of seven days, three mega firms such as Lehman Brothers, Merrill Lynch and AIG declared bankruptcy, ceased to exist as independent entities or needed a massive government bailout. Lehman went insolvent, Merrill was absorbed by Bank of America, and AIG, the insurance giant supposedly with 1 trillion dollars in assets, required a gargantuan government loan of $85 billion. The world was aghast at the week's drama, but watched the events helplessly, because global share markets were in a free fall — yet again.

The main culprit for the current financial mess is Maestro Greenspan. Presidents and Congress were also responsible to a lesser extent because of their intervention in the markets and the economy. There was a report on the Drudge website during that tumultuous week that we were only about 50 trades away from total collapse that could have brought the sale of $250 billion worth of shares. If that had happened, DJIA would have fallen from over 11,000 to possibly below 8,000, a drop of 27 per cent in a day. However, the market did crash later, going below 7,000 due to the uncertainty caused by several reasons, including, as some suggested, the election of Barak Obama as the first black president.

Greenspan's first offence in the early 1980s was to advise the Reagan administration to increase social security taxes on working people and use these funds to lower the deficit as described in detail by Professor Ravi Batra in his book, *Greenspan's Fraud*. Batra believes that this may be one of the most significant causes of the shrinking middle class, leading to greater polarisation in America. Fed Chairman Paul Volcker (1978-87) succeeded in bringing down the inflation rate and should have been reappointed. However, he was replaced by Greenspan, thanks to the latter's political skills. The real estate lobby and Wall Street were against Volcker due to his very tight monetary policy. Some Republicans believe that Greenspan sided with the Democrats to defeat George H.W. Bush by tightening money supply that caused a recession in 1991-92. If this is true, he is more of a politician than an economist, as Batra claims.

Where Greenspan bears the biggest responsibility is in creating the era of cheap money policy that spawned two speculative bubbles. He created them in spite of the fact that he was warned of the risks. He even acknowledged the potential danger of his policy through his famous *irrational exuberance* speech in 1996, but did not do anything about it. He could have brought some control by increasing the margin requirement for the purchase of shares. He was warned a second time in 1998 by the Commodity Future Trading Commission about the explosive rise in derivative instruments described by Warren Buffet as "investment instruments of mass destruction". Please note that these derivative products also include sub-prime mortgages. Greenspan was against any new regulation arguing that it would disrupt the capital markets.

With no move to keep any control, share prices went up to the moon in 1999 and early 2000, creating a giant tech bubble. As prices rose, brokers increasingly loaned money to the public to buy shares, and prices kept rising until the bubble burst. Then came the misfortune of 9/11. The Dow Jones Index went from about 12,000 to 8,000. "The man who saved the World", Greenspan, knocked down the Fed fund interest rate below one per cent. Bruised by the stock market losses, Americans started to buy and speculate in houses. Wall Street professionals, we know, are experts in creative financing. They came up with instruments like securitised bonds and collateralised debt obligations (CDO). They packaged these instruments at different risk levels and creased a market for them. Greenspan this time got involved in favouring these investments; he would say repeatedly that housing was a safe investment because home prices rarely fall, and if they do, a home owner could wait things out till the price comes back. He even encouraged people to borrow at a variable mortgage rate, which is quite risky. Greenspan dismissed the argument that a new bubble was emerging. He would describe it as "froth" in a few areas. Later, when investments in CDOs started to fall apart in 2007-08, he conceded that the word "bubble" should have been used in place of "froth". When froth keeps accumulating, it evolves into an ever expanding bubble. It is amazing that no one in financial markets, Congress, or the Bush government saw the problem associated with wildly imprudent lending to anyone, creditworthy or not. It is pure lunacy to lend to totally unworthy applicants by assigning finite risk when we know that the risk could be infinite. The bankers did it by creating subprime mortgages — meaning lower creditworthiness than prime — and variable interest rates.

Alan Greenspan, as Fed chairman, was a regulator of the banking industry for almost two decades. Federal Reserve, as an institution, is responsible for maintaining sound money policies so that inflation and interest rates are in control. In 2002, he was knighted by the British Queen for promoting "economic stability". Six years later, markets were gyrating as if the world was coming to an end; AIG, the largest insurance company, Fannie Mae, and Freddie Mac, the largest mortgage companies, had in effect been nationalised to avoid financial catastrophe. The government spent 1 trillion dollars so that the cancer created by subprime mortgages did not kill the banking industry. Greenspan describes this "Black Swan" event as the one that occurs "once in a hundred years". I would describe Greenspan himself as a "Black Swan", and a politician of politicians gifted with unusual communication skills. Please note that a "Black Swan" is a highly unpredictable and unquantifiable event that carries a massive impact.

The previous chapter gave you a brief account of some well-known schools of thought that have appeared since ancient times. However, modern economics dates back to Adam Smith's masterpiece, the *Wealth of Nations*, which appeared in 1776. Over two centuries have passed since the publication of that work, and although many schools and sub-schools now exist in economics, they can all be divided in three categories. Thus, basically there are three schools — interventionist, non-interventionist and hybrid or the mixed economy. The interventionists hold that the government should lend a helping hand to keep an otherwise free enterprise system stable by means of monetary and fiscal policies. Financial institutions should be tightly regulated, anti-trust laws should be duly enforced to maintain keen competition among firms and industries, the minimum wage should be indexed to prices, and so on. The chief mentor of interventionists is Keynes and his followers, the neo-Keynesians.

The non-interventionist school, by contrast, believes that there should be no minimum wage and the markets should be left alone, that the government should be lax even in the matter of anti-trust laws, and that the economy is the most efficient when the government stays out of people's financial decisions. In this view, the private sector tends to heal itself and defeats any crisis with its own flexibility. It is somewhat like homoeopathic medicine, where the operating principle is that the body is prompted to take care of itself without any external intervention. The chief proponent of non-interventionists is Joseph Schumpeter, the one who relies on creative destruction of capitalism to be actually a healing process. The mixed-economy school grudgingly accepts the minimum wage and argues that the markets should be left alone until there is a crisis afflicting Wall Street and big companies; at that point, the government should intervene and use taxpayers' money to rescue the major companies. Some firms, in this view, are too big and important to fail. It is the mixed or the hybrid school that, under the tutelage of trickle-down or supply-side economists, has shaped government policy since the early 1980s, when Ronald Reagan became president.

The Sway of the Hybrid School

The mixed-economy school acted in full blast during the stock market crash of 2008, when the Dow Jones Index fell over 40 per cent from its peak reached on 9 October 2008. The government spent ½ trillion dollars to bail out Wall Street firms such as Bear Stearns, Fannie Mae, Freddie Mac and AIG to shore up the stock market and when that did not help, it engineered another bailout of $800 billion in the month of September, this time to rescue virtually the entire Wall Street. The officials argued that their intervention was necessary to protect the financial system from collapse. These were the same people who had detested government involvement in business matters all their life. They had remained quiet when Wall Street was raking in money with its complex and risky schemes used in an orgy of speculation; they had been silent even when oil prices broke record after record from that speculation and the public suffered. But when the share market turned sour, the officials relented and turned the US economy systematically into corporate socialism. Even CNBC and Fox News Channel, the chief media for disseminating the views of the mixed-economy school, felt outraged by the immense government bailouts of the administration and branded its policy as socialism. The main proponents of this school are Alan Greenspan and now the current Fed chairman, Ben Bernanke. It abhors Keynesian thought but regularly puts into practice neo-Keynesian policies, whenever Wall Street profits and bonuses are threatened.

After Bear Stearns was saved from bankruptcy, Martin Wolf, of the *Financial Times*, London, wrote, "This is the day the dream of global free-market capitalism died."

The Federal Reserve now intervenes in any financial institution in one way or another. It has probably become the most powerful arm of the government. So here comes the fifth branch. The executive branch, seeking to keep the people employed (analogous to the human body), the legislative branch wanting to keep spending money (analogous to human emotions), the judiciary, seeking to implement the laws (analogous to human intellect and reasoning), and the undeclared branch, the media, which provides information and influences public opinion (analogous to human genetics, the human blueprint); and finally, the Federal Reserve, the all-encompassing saviour of all, the Absolute, providing cash to make sure that the economic machinery does not fall apart.

Economics is not a science; economists try hard to argue like physicists and make nature a slave of science. Economics is closely connected to human psychology and therefore, to nature. Recall the rule that hindsight is 20/20 but nature is 80/20. We try to predict tsunamis and earthquakes, but with little success. Humanity has taken Nature's rule of 80/20 in many different ways. Nature's non-linear functioning is applied to leveraged investments that give leveraged profit.

However, leveraging is like a double-edged sword, as it can also wipe out your investment. Violent fluctuations, seen in markets, result often due to a high degree of leveraging. Investment instruments like options, also known as derivatives, are leveraged investments.

The reason Bear Starns was saved was because if it failed, the so-called "side effect" to the entire system would have been disastrous. The current economic system is a system of entanglement due to the complexity caused by derivates. There is a belief among experts that in saving Wall Street from Wall Street, the Fed is taking the right action, since Wall Street has become the beating heart of the financial system. The real economy, spanning from the centres of technology, manufacturing and retail shopping malls, is now so intertwined with the electronic bits and paper economy that a disaster on Wall Street spreads like a fire spreading from the heart towards the peripheral economic body.

A lot of "Flation" occurred in 2008. Flation? Yes, deflation took place in housing and financial assets including long-term junk bonds. However inflation occurred in food, oil, and the metals. And for years, we know that the value of labour in the Western economy has been going down, thanks to cheap labour in Asia. We need a miracle to bring back the balance of the two pairs of economic opposites; the four elements of two pairs are GDP growth, unemployment rate, the interest rate and the inflation rate.

This brings us to the current state of economics, especially macroeconomics. While numerous schools of thought and three broad categories exist in economics, unfortunately none of them explains what has been happening in the US and around the world since 1980. Here are some of the events that beg for analysis and understanding:

1. Why are governments around the world, including USA, sinking in a sea of debt?

2. Why are American families drowning in debt?
3. Why did profits first surge all over the world in the 2000s, then crashed, and then surge again in 2009 and 2010 even as 20 million people remained jobless in the US?
4. Why are there frequent stock market bubbles and crashes in recent years?
5. Why did the housing industry experience an all-time high bubble?
6. Why did the housing market crash and a credit crisis ensue?
7. Why do trade deficits and surpluses persist in the globe?
8. Why did the international price of oil hit an all-time record in 2008, then collapsed, and soared again?
9. What are the real causes of unemployment, recessions and depressions?

The schools of thought explored so far deal with only question no. 9; they don't even tackle the other puzzles, let alone explain them. Is there any theory that can singly analyse all the questions raised above? Fortunately, there is one thesis that rises to this challenge, and that is the theory of the wage gap offered by Professor Batra. Batra first expounded this idea in his 1999 book, *The Crash of the Millennium*, and then explored it further in three other books, *Common Sense Macroeconomics, Greenspan's Fraud,* and *The New Golden Age*. In another article appearing in a book edited by Professor Rajani Kanth, Batra simplified the wage gap theory even further to make it easier to understand, and tackled the questions listed above, and the presentation here mostly relies on this latest version. An article by Kendall Anderson in *Fort Worth Weekly* also deals with the concept of the wage gap, making it easier to follow.

The wage gap theory is astoundingly simple, and yet it tackles all the queries posed above. It is indeed remarkable that what numerous economic schools fail to elucidate is explained by one idea, which may be properly called the unified theory of economics. The unified theory of economics offered by Batra is similar to the grand idea of the unified theory of physics in science

The Theory of the Wage Gap

Batra begins with a simple notion. He says that a healthy economy requires a balance between two forces — supply and demand. In a macro system, we, of course, have to examine these forces at the national level. Thus, macroeconomic balance occurs when

$$\text{Supply} = \text{Demand}$$

This balance is very important for a sound economy and prosperity, because if supply exceeds demand, there is overproduction and hence layoffs, and if supply is less than demand, there is high inflation. Up to this point, Batra's position is the same as that of any other school. But now comes the simple but major point of departure. The main source of supply is labour productivity, while the main source of demand is people's wages. Here Batra differs from all other schools, which argue that national output or supply depends on capital, labour and technology, so that supply arises from three sources, not one. But Batra seems to suggest that capital and technology affect production through their impact on productivity, whereas the quality of the labour force does not change much in the short run. In any case, as Batra points out, these other factors can be easily incorporated into his analysis without altering the main conclusions. They just make the analysis more cumbersome, without changing the main thesis.

As regards to demand, the real wage or the average purchasing power of people's wages, is the main source of consumer demand. Here Batra differs substantially from Keynes, neo-Keynesians and other schools that hold that real income, not just the real wage, determines the level of national demand. But the real wage is the main source of demand and that is incontrovertible; it is well known that consumer spending is about 70 per cent of GDP or national demand in the US, and the real wage is the most important factor here.

Since productivity grows over time due to new investment and technology, wages must rise in the same proportion to maintain the demand-supply balance in a natural way. If this does not happen, a wage-productivity gap, or simply a wage gap, develops and the supply-demand balance can be achieved only through government intervention in an artificial way that not only lowers the general standard of living, but also sows the seeds of vast problems in the future. If productivity growth exceeds wage growth, then supply exceeds demand, and overproduction results. Companies have to lay off their workers, which in turn raises unemployment and causes a nightmare for elected officials, who then have two choices. Either they follow policies that raise wages or they follow policies that raise debt, because new debt also creates demand, but in an artificial way. From the 1950s to the 1970s, wages in the US went up nearly as fast as productivity, and the demand supply balance was maintained in a natural way. But, since 1980, wages have been stagnant, and the government has resorted to the creation of debt. It has vastly expanded its budget deficit, calling it fiscal policy. It has also cut interest rates periodically, calling it monetary policy, so people will borrow more money. But whether you call it fiscal or monetary policy, both measures generate new debt in the economy. Since productivity rises every year, debt has to grow exponentially over time to preserve the demand supply balance. This way the economic balance is maintained, but many unintended consequences follow from the rise in the wage gap. These consequences are the same as the first eight questions raised above.

The Global Sea of Debt

The whole world is awash in debt today, especially the governments of most nations. Regardless of how high or low their economic growth has been in recent years, governments worldwide have had huge budget deficits and mountains of debt. In the US, Australia and Canada, even the consumers and some firms are in hawk and have to use a large portion of their income to service their past borrowings. All these are the results of the so-called monetary and fiscal policies that helped raise national demand to national supply and avoided overproduction and hence layoffs. So these policies were dictated by the rising wage gap; otherwise, high joblessness would have occurred and elected officials would have been thrown out. In fact, the US now borrows over $2 billion everyday from abroad to keep its economy functioning.

Vastness of Profits

Greenspan is very fond of explaining the giant profits of companies since 1990 by focusing on large productivity gains that have resulted due to computers and the Internet. The gain in the corporate profit is the result of not just productivity gains but debt growth as well. In the absence of the debt rise, increased production resulting from increased productivity cannot be sold to consumers with stagnant wages. Profit will then fall, rather than rise. High supply alone does not guarantee a profit; the supply has to find buyers as well. Hence the vast growth in debt along with productivity explains the vast rise in profits between 1990 and 2007, and in 2009 and 2010.

Stock Market Bubbles and Crashes

When profits rise sharply, share price bubbles are inevitable. It may be noted that there were no such bubbles during the

1950s and 1960s, when wages kept pace with productivity; nor was there much rise in government and consumer debt. Thus the rise in the wage gap along with debt explains why stock market bubbles have been frequent between 1980 and 2007. But debt cannot rise forever, and the moment it stops increasing, supply exceeds demand, goods go unsold and profits crash. The stock market crashes as well. Thus, the wage gap idea also elucidates the frequent occurrence of stock market bubbles and crashes between 1980 and 2007. The bubbles were busted in 1987, in 2000-01 and then again in 2008.

The Housing Bubble and Crash

How do we explain the housing bubble that occurred between 2001 and 2006? How does the wage gap idea become relevant here? This bubble is not related to company profits, but to Greenspan's policy of slashing some interest rates below 1 per cent. The stock market crash followed by a severe bear market of 2000-02 was so bad that the world feared the onset of a depression. Then Greenspan panicked and brought the interest rates down in a hurry so as to lure the public into even more borrowing. This way he postponed large-scale unemployment, but sowed the seeds of a housing bubble as well as a credit bubble by the banks. Most people buy homes on credit, and when the cost of credit declines dramatically, home demand must soar, leading to a vast rise in home building and jobs in the construction industry. Thus Greenspan was able to postpone the depression, but since debt cannot grow forever, he created the conditions for economic collapse that started in 2007, when some home-buyers began to default on their mortgages. The debt pile that had been building since 1981 turned into a mountain by 2007. And the mountain began to unravel, at first slowly and then at a furious pace. All this led to the failure of several large banks and financial firms on Wall Street. They shed workers, so joblessness began to rise. Banks suffered further losses from their stock investments.

Stung by these losses, they curtailed their lending. That hurt the auto industry, as low-wage consumers were unable to purchase cars. Thus the economy began to unravel like the dominoes. By the end of 2008, a full-fledged and deep recession had set in. The new Fed chairman, Ben Bernanke, applied the same old remedy of cutting interest rates to bare minimum, but this time it failed. People could not increase their borrowings, because their home equity had been used up already; banks were no longer risk-prone as they had suffered huge losses. So the root cause of the credit crunch is again the high wage gap.

China's Trade Surplus

How does the wage gap idea explain giant trade surpluses in countries like China and Japan? When the wage gap rises, supply goes up faster than demand. Then the debt has to rise, both at the consumer and the government level, to absorb the annual and relentless growth in supply. In China and Japan consumer debt did not rise much, because people there like to save a large portion of their income. So the other thing that these nations did was to maintain a low official exchange rate so that they could export their extra production abroad. With low consumer demand at home, they had no choice but to follow mercantilist policies wherein a nation wants to maximise its exports and minimises its imports. They, in effect, transferred their low home-demand problem onto foreign nations.

Of course, the high trade surplus from China and Japan meant a high deficit in other nations, especially the US and the Euro-zone. The deficit nations had high home demand because of vast consumer borrowing resulting from record low interest rates, even though their wage gap had risen. In fact, the purchase of US government bonds by China and Japan kept these interest rates so low that the US home demand exceeded its supply even though its wage gap soared. Thus the root cause of global trade imbalances is also the rising wage gap in the trade surplus nations like China and Japan. If the wage gap had been stable in these countries, their production would have been purchased by their own consumers, thus avoiding the need for artificially low-valued exchange rates and hence the trade surpluses. Absent their surpluses, the rest of the world would not have trade deficits. Thus, the apparent cause of such imbalances are the artificial exchange rates, but the true cause is the growing wage gap in mercantilist nations.

The Oil Bubble and Crash

It is now clear that there was an oil bubble as well in 2008, as the oil price hit $147 per barrel in July and then collapsed to less than $40 by the end of the year. In *The New Golden Age*, written in 2006, Batra had actually predicted the rise of this bubble and then a crash in 2009, although he missed the crash period by about six months. Yet he was one of the few who had forecast oil's steep rise and then collapse. There were others, such as T. Boone Pickens and Mathew Simmons, who predicted an oil shortage for decades to come, with the price approaching as high as $200. Financial firms such as Goldman Sachs and Morgan Stanley that were heavily speculating in oil were also in their camp, arguing that rising oil demand from high growth nations such as India and China created a global shortage of oil. Even Greenspan saw the rise in oil as a natural result of rising economic growth from India and China. But then from July on oil prices began to crash even though India and China still exist and their oil appetite is still more or less is the same as before. As usual, the Maestro toed the line of big business and was clearly wrong.

Where does the wage gap idea fit in the oil boom and bust? When productivity rises but wages do not, then profits soar with the help of soaring debt, and these profits chase speculative activities, because opportunities for business expansion remain constrained by limited consumer demand. So speculation abounds in all types of markets, including housing, commodities and shares. If the wage gap had been constant, profits would not have risen sharply, and then speculation would be limited. The rising wage gap along with debt always leads to high profits and the proliferation of risky ventures that misfire in the end.

Then why did oil price collapse? The reason is the same that punctures all bubbles eventually. When the credit flow stops, and/or the money supply shrinks, bubbles end. Once the banks began to lose money from their soured mortgage-backed securities and then suffered losses in share markets, they reduced their lending to oil speculators as well. With the flow of funds curtailed, oil buying went down, and so did its price. The oil price had to collapse, especially in a recessionary environment all over the world.

The Real Cause of Unemployment and Recessions

Keynesian economics explains unemployment by means of the lack of demand relative to supply. But the shortage of demand arises from a rise in inequality. As inequality rises, the rich get richer and save a lot more than the poor and the middle class. So the savings of the rich tend to rise, leading to a fall in consumer demand and hence in employment. The average American is not saving anymore. The savings rate in the US has been practically zero for a long time; so why is consumer demand low relative to product supply? Keynesian economics cannot answer this question by claiming a high level of savings, which are actually very low. The only explanation is that supply is now rising faster than demand because of the rising wage gap and since debt growth has slowed, there is overproduction, leading to mounting layoffs.

Two million workers lost jobs in 2008 alone, and 2009 witnessed more job losses, with both General Motors and Chrysler declaring bankruptcy. The companies did survive but not without a $50 billlion bailout. According to Wall Street and government economists, the "Great Recession" ended in mid-2009, but job losses continued for months thereafter. If you include discouraged workers, who are excluded from the definition of the labour force, the unemployment rate was as high as 15 per cent even at the start of 2010. Since wages continue to stagnate, there will be little rise in consumer demand. However, productivity growth is not likely to slow, because of further automation. Consequently, the supply-demand gap will only expand in the future. So we should expect high joblessness for many years to come. It is indeed remarkable that Batra's unified theory of economics explains all the nine questions posed above. No wonder Thom Hartmann, the celebrated host of the Thom Hartmann Show on Air America, and Kendall Anderson, a journalist, compare Batra's theories with those of the heretic like John Maynard Keynes.

Nature and the Wage Gap Theory

In his book, *Basic Economics,* Thomas Sowell convincingly argues that laws of economics, like the law of demand and supply, work best when there is minimum government interference. Economic laws are comparable to the laws of nature. Freedom of choice extends the life of an entity, including organisms and organisations. A healthy heart, or any organ of an organism, functions well if there is no external intrusion like poking a knife or shooting a bullet into it. This is true for every natural system that keeps functioning autonomously throughout its lifespan; Mother Earth will keep rotating around the sun and the sun will rise and set far beyond our own existence.

The supply and demand are linked to the labour market, via productivity and wages. We can demonstrate that in order to ensure minimum government interference in the economy, wages should keep up with productivity; otherwise, supply rises faster than demand and government intervention in the form of debt creation becomes indispensable to avoid layoffs. Thus the message here, though similar to Sowell's, offers a prescription, namely the government should avoid policies that raise the wage-productivity gap. In other words, the *laisséz faire* approach works well if there is enough competition among firms for workers so that wages rise with productivity. This means that the anti-trust laws have to be fully enforced so that competition remains intense and merger-related layoffs are avoided.

Nature and the 80/20 Rule

As stated in an earlier chapter, Nature's favourite sport is to create pairs of opposites for the purpose of their mutual survival. The 80/20 principle shows that Nature is often non-linear and how survival through the coexistence of opposites becomes possible. The principle states that 80 per cent of a task is relatively easy and can be done in 20 per cent of the time; the remaining 20 per cent of the task is difficult and can take the remaining 80 per cent of the time. The 80/20 principle also implies that work gets harder as one approaches the completion of the task. This principle was first discovered in 1897 by the Italian economist Vilfredo Pareto. Living in the nineteenth-century England, Pareto found that 80 per cent of wealth and income in Britain went to just 20 per cent of people, a small minority. The same is true in the US today.

The 80/20 principle was rediscovered by Harvard professor George Zipf in 1944; he called it the Principle of Least Effort. There are numerous examples of the 80/20 phenomenon in our lives. For example, 20 per cent of motorists cause 80 per cent of accidents; 20 per cent of those who get married comprise 80 percent of divorce statistics. This figure implies that the statistic of a 40 per cent divorce rate in America (4 out of 10) is actually deceiving. It is more accurate to say that two couples out of 10 get divorced, not once, but twice, increasing the divorce rate artificially to 40 per cent. Examples of the 80-20 relationship are so frequent that it may be called an integral law of nature.

Adi Shankara, some 12 centuries ago, advised us that to learn more about a nemesis, the learner should become one with the latter's way of thinking. This advice implies that a nemesis is the opposition or competition, not necessarily an enemy to destroy. Shankara's thesis tells us that a pair of opposites must learn to coexist in balance, harmony and complement each other for the greater good. Living organisms coexist in multidimensional space to survive. Multiple pairs of opposites constitute multidimensional space. In an unpredictable Nature, multiple pairs of opposites must exist to maintain life. Elements of a pair of opposites cannot be separated, anymore than the north pole of a magnet can be separated from the south pole. Ancient Vedic teachers would say that these two opposites need to complement each other instead of being at war so that they can coexist in balance and harmony.

In short, pairs of opposites must coexist for survival. Using the 80/20 principle found in Nature, we can create a better economy, raise our living standard, and aid our survival as human beings. A marriage of a man and woman is probably the most well-known example of opposites coexisting, and from it comes society's fabric. The husband and wife must learn to coexist and thrive in marriage. They must learn to complement each other and not compete, as though one might be the nemesis of the other. If they successfully do so, they will most likely have a successful life with loving and successful children. If parents don't coexist successfully, their children will suffer and bring those scars back into society. As India's imminent physicist, J. Bose, says, "Learn, respect, and love Nature — Nature probably will help you put on the right path of life".

Similarly, business executives and their workers must learn to coexist in harmony, equally share in the fruit of rising productivity, and not look upon each other as adversaries. Batra's wage gap theory accords with the 80/20 principle. In fact, the history of the 1950s and the 1960s shows that healthy economic growth follows this rule. In those decades US economic growth was exceptionally strong — varying between 4 and 4.5 per cent per year. These were also the decades when labour's share of national income was 80 per cent and capital's share was 20 per cent — exactly in line with the 80/20 rule. Wages and productivity then went up together, and did so in much of US history. Since 1980, however, labour's share has fallen to 70 per cent while capital's share has risen to 30 per cent, thereby violating the natural rule, and not surprisingly growth has been slow, averaging 3 per cent. Moreover, economic growth during the 2000s was just 2 per cent per year, mostly because of the Great Recession.

We can reflect on the 80/20 rule that constitutes many examples of opposites coexisting. There is evidently a good side as well as a bad side of the principle, as is clear from the wage gap theory. The good side is that when wages and productivity rose together, as from 1950 to 1970, so that labour's share remained high and constant, then the US economy flourished for all and everyone prospered. The governmental intervention in the economy was also minimal at that time. But when this rule was violated so that we faced its opposite with 20 per cent possessing 80 per cent of wealth, then the living standards began to decline for the vast majority of people, and the government became more intrusive, so much so that in 2008 it followed the principles of socialism and bought stake in many financial firms. The moral is that a good economy ought to follow the good side of the 80/20 rule. We should not be at a point where the economy cannot grow without trillions of dollars in new government debt.

5

Clustering, Balance, Harmony and Complementarities

Clustering and Unity within the Diversity of Four

CLUSTERING is a natural tendency. A tribal man is lost when he is away from his tribe. The majority of people prefer to be part of a group. Grouping is universal. However, one does not need to be attached to groups, since in order to enter into the spiritual domain and merge with Universal Consciousness, there must be detachment from worldly matters

An analogy might be helpful. Driving on a four- or five-lane freeway in a place like California, one comes across clusters of cars, formed through speed limits. The "nature" of the freeway, its many lanes, speed limits, and so on, produces clusters "naturally," but the "enlightened" driver would stay out of such clusters to lower the probability of accidents with other cars. In the field of investment, it may be less profitable to be part of a herd. Often, contrarians receive better returns on their investment.

I recall a game we played as children on weekends and holidays in the 1940s in India, before independence — Mahatma Gandhi's Non-Violent Resistance Movement (Satyagraha). Kids would get together in clusters, acting as freedom fighters. The objective for everyone was to get into a one-metre-square-sized area on the grass, called "the jail." The jail space would be a few feet away from about 25 kids who competed. Winners were those found in the square at the end of ten minutes. Smaller kids would not attempt to get into jail, since it was hard to compete with bigger and stronger kids. If I stayed with kids of my size, I could never get into jail. However, when I made an attempt, I succeeded in getting in the jail by finding a void, a little space for little me among the bigger kids. I was the happiest "contrarian" small kid to be part of a cluster of "giant" winners.

We all remember phrases like, "When it rains, it pours," or "Nature is always unpredictable, like fish swimming here and there with sudden twists and turns," or, more romantically, "Women are unpredictable, like autumn skies." What do such utterances really say beyond their surface meaning? I would suggest that these sayings indicate the significance and structure of clustering. Clustering is a non-uniform, uneven distribution of elements or events. It is a characteristic feature of Nature, as observed in the clustering of stars and planets. At the micro-level, the simple but lifesaving process of blood clotting in a wound is an instance of clustering. At the macro-level events occur in clusters, good and bad. Clustering is the cause of likes, dislikes, hate crimes, tribalism, empire building and one of the Kennedy brothers in the Senate for over fifty years. President George W. Bush became unpopular because so many unfortunate events occurred during his presidency though he was not responsible for some of them. These patterns occur also in the marketplace, in the movement of prices in the stock market, indicating the mass psychology of the stock traders. Clusters are therefore, not only material but also psychic patterns. This gives one more evidence that psychic selves are associated with Nature, like somatic selves.

Based on this, I will now introduce a special, basic pattern of clustering, occurring in two pairs, and four elements.

There is already so much in the world that is divided into threes, starting with the basic division of many things as having a beginning, middle and end. Certainly the Hindu Trinity of Brahma, Vishnu and Shiva finds some parallel in the Catholic Trinity of Father, Son and Holy Spirit. Jonah spent three days in the belly of a whale and Jesus spent three days in his tomb. One could also think of clusters of five — for example, there are five fingers, five basic elements, five gods in Hindu tradition, and five Ajivas in the Jain tradition. We could go on and on, but in our embracing three or five as a classic archetype, we have overlooked a more common occurrence of the number four. There are, after all, four seasons, four corners of the world, and four winds. If we look even closer, we can see that four, the number of stability, which can also be represented by two pairs of opposite or similar things, is perhaps the most common numeral in much of our daily life.

To begin our numerical study of the number four, we need to recognise that ancient Indians divided human existence into three autonomous domains, namely somatic, psychic, and spiritual. Western thinkers originally divided existence into three levels of Heaven, Hell and Earth. The first two levels (somatic and psychic), associated with Nature, are also models for the number four, if we limit our focus to the natural part of our being that includes somatic and psychic levels and investigate their interrelationships and transcendence.

Firstly, Nature itself exists in multiple pairs of opposites. The four seasons of spring, summer, fall and winter certainly form two pairs. Interestingly, these multiple pairs of opposites are also found within man himself. They are pairs that cannot be separated (for example, the north pole of a magnet cannot be separated from the south pole). These two opposites, ancient Indians would say, need to "complement" each other instead of being at war, so that they can coexist in balance and harmony.

The recent application of the word "complementarity" was introduced by the quantum physicist Niels Bohr. His observations were based on the discovery of subatomic particles such as electrons behaving as particles and waves (a pair of opposites). Bohr showed us that at the deepest levels of physical reality, things are not definitely spotty or smooth. This ambiguity is a result of neither vagueness nor contradiction, but Nature itself. An analogous situation can be described about a human person as a distinct individual or a nexus in the web of social interaction.

The implication of the principle of complementarity is that a person is both an individual and a social component (another pair of opposites), and there is no need to separate the two. On a philosophical level, we can say that reality is "One" (Universal Self), and language is really its opposite, because it introduces unnecessary distinctions that need not be made. Bohr's strong belief in complementarity led him to make a singular statement: "A great truth is a statement whose opposite is also a great truth." Recall comparing the truth with the beauty of many facets of a diamond or the story of the blind men of Hindustan and an elephant by the sages of India, thousands of years ago.

Robert Oppenheimer, a physicist who led a team of scientists to develop the first nuclear bomb, tried to convince the world that sciences and humanities are a pair of opposites; they complement each other and are not disconnected. He may have come to this conclusion based on his studies of Vedic scriptures in the original Sanskrit language.

Adi Shankara in the eighth century stated: become a detached witness to learn about and understand nemesis. Even try to become "the other" in order to understand the opposite. Let us ask, what is this "opposite"? Pairs of opposites could coexist in balance and harmony if we learned to become detached witnesses, as preached by Shankara. Pairs of opposites could complement each other for a common cause. Take an example of a married couple. Husband and wife can compete and fight with each other, which can be destructive, or they could complement each other, maintaining balance and harmony with a result of better life for them and their children.

The number four, in modern times, comes centrestage through psychologist Carl Jung's work when he describes fundamental patterns of human thought not as dyad but tetrad, that is, two pairs of opposites having a total of four elements in a balanced mandala-like arrangement, also known as "quaternary." Jung describes the quaternary as an archetype of almost universal occurrence. It forms the logical basis for any whole judgement; if one wishes to pass such a judgement, it must have this fourfold aspect. There are always four elements, four prime qualities, four castes, four ways of spiritual development, and four aspects of psychic orientation. The ideal of completeness is the circle of a sphere, but its natural minimal division is quaternary. Note that Jung talks about four castes and four ways of spiritual development, evidently influenced by Indian philosophy, which he may have discovered during his visit to India.

Jung describes the human body in four parts — sensation (body), feeling (emotion), thinking (intellect), and intuition (mind). His understanding of intuition includes something other than or beyond sensation, feeling and thinking. I interpret it to be associated with the initial condition of human existence, that is, genetics in the realm of human equipment. Perhaps I am taking a leap when I say that evolutionary change occurred during human history in four stages.

During the first stage, there was greater emphasis on the body and associated elements. The second stage was that of the mind. Then came an emphasis on the intellect. And the latest stage was the age of information and genetics. Based on our observation of life, it does not de-emphasise the fact that there are four stages to it, just as there are four elements (fire, air, water, earth) and four points on a compass (north, south, east, and west). Spiritually, recall that Buddhism had four Noble Truths and Christianity celebrates four Gospels that were actually mandated by a second-century book by St. Irenaeus, *Against the Heresies*, where the Eastern author pronounces the number four as being sanctioned by Nature itself in the four winds.

However, I would like to emphasise that Nature exists in multi-dimensions, and within each pair of dimensions are two opposites. These pairs cannot be separated and each pair coexists with all the others. If we take this as a model of the total human self, we can conclude that one needs to learn to complement the opposites of oneself, and not be at war with oneself. By evolving and adapting to our changing environment, complementary pairs of opposites bring balance and harmony to our lives and help us to coexist with others. We can also realise that all four elements make up the whole with no one element being inferior or superior to the others, each one equal and coexistent, with its own autonomy and freedom.

A few additional examples are in order. Cluster formations are natural phenomena. Recall at the mega-level that stars form clusters in the cosmos; at the micro-level, blood-clotting happens in the human body; at the macro-level the old boys' club becomes the corporate world; Indians cluster in Little India; and so on. An organisation, a form of a cluster, tends to become stagnant. If the CEO is not careful, it could stop evolving to higher levels or stop sub-rating. Organisations are almost always hierarchical. Leaders try to hold to their positions at the expense of the organisation.

Detachment is more helpful to sub-rate, transcend, and move upward toward the mountaintop. Institutional hierarchies tend to generate empire builders and protectors who persecute those who do not fall in line. Living organisms exist in multidimensional space as multiple pairs of opposites. Organisms must find and exist at locations away from boundaries; they perish if they hit a boundary. It is necessary to maintain balance in a space with two pairs of opposites and four boundaries of quaternaries, as suggested by Jung and the ancient sages of India. Recall Buddha's message of the Middle Path of existence.

Different quaternaries are given at the end of this chapter. The four elements of the total human self are connected to the four elements in different fields described by ancient Indian masters, mathematicians and physicists.

> **Note**: Separations of opposites of each pair, in each category in the tables, are not unique, and cannot be exact. The process of separation and the identification of the four are debatable and changeable, as happens in Nature. Identification often becomes difficult when we do not know what we are trying to separate or when there are too many variables.

More on Multidimensional Space

On matters of multidimensional space constituted by pairs of opposites, deeper explanation is required. We exist in this space, but our existence is dynamic. It has to be — it cannot be stagnant; nature demands it. The characteristics of this space keep changing in time and we must adjust our position in this space to survive and prosper. For most of us, we need to find the sweet spot in the middle of the space of our existence and try to occupy as close as we can get to it. Dynamic changes create fluctuations, like the movement of a pendulum, but not necessarily at constant frequencies and amplitude. These movements are complex and mathematicians have tried to make these movements deterministic but with very limited success. Books have been written with titles like *Deterministic*

Chaos, etc. to prosper in various markets. No computer can solve such multidimensional problems accurately since the nature within and without is unpredictable. However, humanity has learnt a lot through experience and with the use of intellect and intuition. We have achieved limited success simplifying every problem. For example, talking about the movements of the pendulum, analogically we can find the frequencies, periods and displacement of these fluctuations. We would also know where and when the pendulum stops and changes its direction of movement. We also know that it spends the longest time at the location where it changes its direction and the least (minimum) time at the middle of the swing where the speed is the highest. Movements are necessary to be dynamic, to be alive. When we are talking about an organic life form, the heart has to keep beating, blood has to keep flowing. We are also dependent, for example, on the movements of the earth; it has to keep orbiting, but movements must be orderly, without hitting the boundaries of the space of our existence.

Guide to the Table

The table at the end of the chapter is self-explanatory by nature and structure. The table leads us to observe fully a remarkable spectrum of the correspondence between the four aspects of Nature and the four domains of the total human self. Furthermore, there is also a correspondence between the four domains of the total human self and the four branches of mathematics; the four aspects of economics and political power; the four stages of life; the four systems of human motives; and several other sets of four.

In order to understand these tables, let us first note the categories that form their structure. They are: Nature; Total human self; any specific field of their interaction, for example, mathematics or the four branches of government, and so on.

The four aspects of Nature are: Cosmic Order; Earth and Matter; Ākāśa or Space, which is continuous and spacious; and Time, which is unidirectional, that is, thermodynamic and dynamic (See Summary of Tables and Table 1, row 5).

The four domains of the total human self that interact with these four aspects of Nature are first, the DNA of the somatic self, which can be related to the origin — seeds (Bijatma), sperm or egg. The body of the somatic self (Dehatma) includes the heart, brain, and other parts of the body. The intuitive mind of the psychic self has the attributes of love (Prematma), devotion, belief, and the idealism of the philosophic self. The intellectual aspect of the psychic self has the attributes of reasoning, control, and other intellectual capabilities (Gyanatma) (See Tables 1 to 5, row 1, and Summary of Tables).

The four branches of the foundational science of mathematics are: the theory of information, arithmetic, geometry, and algebra/calculus.

All items in the first column of all five tables are associated with genetics. We have seen how the theory of information with its dots corresponds to the genetic blueprint, with its seeds and drops. The information implies that there is stored potential energy in blueprints. They are also the initial conditions of order coming out of chaos that will progress in the future. The initial condition of investment is the initial capital to be invested in any enterprise. Information is also associated with the news media, the supplier of information, considered the fourth branch of the government. The initial creative idea goes a long way to provide a very high growth rate in any start-up enterprise.

Items associated with the body of the somatic self are given in the second column of the table. The body is associated with discrete (digital) matter and organisms, and, considering its functions, actions and attributes, is associated with arithmetic, karma and karma yoga, matter, actions, gravity, employment, Karl Marx, the executive branch of government, and the earth. Autonomy, austerity, and being nonjudgemental are important attributes that the physical body should possess.

Items given in the third column of the table are associated with the intuitive mind of the psychic self, responsible for love, devotion, desires, intuition, spontaneity, spaciousness, and continuity. Geometry deals with specific shapes in space. It measures (metri) earth-spaces (geo). It can be seen that geometry is analogous to the space component of the intuitive mind. Shapes, real estate, and spaciousness are associated with geometry. Determination, compassion, desires, the act of willing, the path of sub-ration, philosophic idealism, transcendence, and a devotional temperament are all attributes of the intuitive mind. The legislative branch of the government prompts the executive branch to run the country's economy with an excessive money supply to maintain a lower unemployment rate.

Items in the fourth and the last column of the table are associated with the intellectual mind of the psychic self. Algebra and calculus deal with certain aspects of temporality. They are analogous to the time components of the intellectual part (Gyanatma) of the psychic self. Intellect brings with it such evolutes as precise logic, logical reasoning, higher intellectual pursuits, as well as discipline and control of both body and mind. Conservative economists are concerned about the value of currency since they believe inflation is not good for people, certainly not retirees and those living on a fixed income. They control inflation by increasing the cost of money, that is, by increasing the interest rate. The function of the judiciary is to maintain law and order and adhere to the nation's constitution. Logical interpretation of the law becomes very important.

Origin, Balance and the Harmony of All

Let us look at the scientific units of measurement and units of the total human self, the former produced and used by the different branches of science, the latter proposed by the author of this book for use in the science or art of what I have called the Samskaric way of individual and global living.

We have learnt about things of Nature through observation, experiences, intellectual thought processes, comparisons, and finally accurate measurements. There are fundamental units of measurement for length, weight, time, temperature, electrical energy, luminosity of light, and so on. We are familiar with such terms as metre and foot; gram and pound; second; ampere; Kelvin, and others. The rest of a unit's measurements are derived from the fundamental units of measurement in each branch of scientific observation. Different combinations of fundamental units provide us with more complex measurements. Thus, for example, velocity is measured in meters (a unit of length) per second (a unit of time); acceleration is determined quantitatively by measuring the change in velocity and is expressed in meters/second squared. Units of energy are obtained by multiplying force with distance or mass multiplied by acceleration multiplied by distance.

I propose taking somatic and psychic units as the basic units of the total human self, to be combined in different ways for our use. The optimum combination, I propose, would be the combination of four. We need to note that genetics and the physical body (from the somatic self) and intuition and intellect (from the psychic self) provide us with the four basic units of our total human self. The rest, which would include any field of human endeavour, can be connected to these primary units. This could be considered as a corollary to physicist Brandon Carter's Anthropic Principle, which states that the only things that can be known are those compatible with the existence of the knowers, the total human selves. From this could be derived the origin, balance and harmony of all.

The two groups in humanity, intellectuals and intuitivists need to be in balance and complement each other to bring harmony. The first group includes materialists and the second group includes religionists. As the population keeps increasing, the needs of the somatic selves keep increasing. It is apparent that the population of materialists keeps increasing. This trend needs to be checked and humanity needs to reverse it. Humanity needs more bridge-builders to bring balance and harmony between intellectuals and intuitivists so that they complement and not compete.

The five tables represent the interconnectedness of everything to the total human self and Nature. They also describe the origin and evolutionary progress of humanity. I re-emphasise that the balance and harmony of the four in a particular field of human endeavour give us optimum results. After dividing the specific field of endeavour into four components, we must ensure that each one operates autonomously without interference.

One of the most successful examples appears to be the American government with their four autonomous components — executive, judiciary, legislative, and the national media, the information provider. It is remarkable that the government has endured assassinations, wars, Watergate, 9/11, and evolved to a level of complexity to minimise the effect of such events. It is not a perfect system of governance, but nothing in Nature is perfect. The most admirable part of the U.S. government appears to be that it is adaptive. In the words of Condoleeza Rice, the U.S. intends to follow the path that leads to "practical idealism." These same two words were uttered by the philosopher-kings of ancient times to uplift their subjects.

Another example is in the field of investment. Harry Markowitz received the Nobel Prize for proving that it is unsafe to put all your eggs in one basket. The implication is that one needs to invest in at least four non-correlating groups of investment to minimise risk. Four non-correlating investments associated with four elements of the total human self are growth stocks, treasuries and monies, real estate and resource stocks, and hard assets like portable gold coins and collectables, as shown in Table 4.

More on the Idea of Balancing the Four

We shall take the example of the current state of the economy (2008), where we are, and what we need to do to improve the situation. The four components in the field of economics, associated with genetics, the body, the intuitive mind, and intellect are: the GDP or economic growth rate, the unemployment rate, inflation rate, and interest rate, respectively. For a good economy, except GDP, all the remaining three components should be lower, possibly below three per cent. Since America is a rich, developed country, any number greater than 3 per cent is acceptable. Let us examine what the current situation is.

On August 21, 2008, I was fortunate to attend a one-time movie event titled, "I.O.U.S.A." shown in 400 U.S. cities to give a critical message to the public. The movie was followed by a live panel discussion. Panel participants included Warren Buffett, CEO of AARP, Bill Novelli, Cato chairman Niskanen, and David M. Walker, former head of Government Accounting Office (GAO) under both the Clinton and Bush presidencies from 1998 to 2008. GAO is nonpartisan and keeps an eye on government spending and reports to Congress. The message from the movie and panel discussion was simple. America is heading toward a financial tsunami if we do not act immediately. We are all familiar with recent problems that include the sub-prime mortgage meltdown, the housing bubble burst, nationalization of Fannie Mae and Freddie Mac, and bailing out the U.S. auto industries. The rising debt problem could accelerate toward the stratosphere. The problem is compounding due to almost zero household savings and uncontrolled consumption, and the rising cost of social security and medical benefits.

The debt could rise to over 50 trillion dollars in a couple of decades if no action is taken. If the projections are accurate, the most menacing culprit will be the rising cost of medical benefits due to the rising population of baby-boomer retirees. Some of the proposed solutions were to increase the retirement age, change tax laws to increase the household savings, and better health management.

America has been on the wrong track ever since we let go of the production economy and went increasingly to a consumption economy. A ball park measure of production is the production of steel. The 19th century belonged to England because they were the largest producers of steel in the world. America was on the top in the 20th century because America was the largest producer of steel. The 21st century seems to belong to China since they are at the top in the same.

There has been a perception that we can maintain our standard of living just by innovation. If we use our minds, we do not have to produce steel or any other hardware in a factory. Some American economists would say about Asia and America that, "we think and they sweat." I would like to counter this by saying, "we must sweat, think, and philosophise" for our well-being. There would be more people earning better wages in manufacturing than those employed in service industries if we were to adopt this course. Wealth is created by producing more, not by consuming more. We should never stop being creative and come up with ideas that give us a better life. The rocket scientists employed by the

Wall Street have done more damage to the financial markets; markets cannot be controlled employing only science. Rocket scientists are trained to solve the problems of technology and not the mind. We must go even further and enter the realm of psychology and philosophy. I believe economic laws have connections to savings, fairness, austerity, and many other human attributes.

More recently, we, have heard about peak oil, peak water, and peak food implying that these commodities will become scarcer in time because the production cannot catch up with consumption. Yes, it is likely that it could happen since more people in Asia would like to have the same lifestyle as those in the West. Then there are two peaks that go hand in hand; they are peak consumption and peak stupidity. Over-consumption is not good for our health; obesity in the West is the highest. Why don't we have peak caution, not peak greed? I suppose greed caused the financial companies to be so highly leveraged. Now we are going into the process of deleveraging. The pendulum is changing the direction from extreme greed and consumption toward caution and hopefully saving for a rainy day.

I hope, some time in the future America will lead the world in climbing the mountain of austerity. Austerity here does not mean ascetic, but simpler living, avoiding waste, living in a smaller house, drive a smaller car, and be environmentally friendly. Climbing a mountain is not an easy endeavour for anyone. America may have to descend a little, go around the obstacles as long as the direction is toward the mountain top. The day America is at the austerity mountain top will be a day to celebrate. We will be in harmony with nature around us, harmony of body, mind, and spirit.

Let us consider the period from October 1st, 2008 through the first week of December 2008. The world is going through a financial tsunami and governments have not been able to establish market stability. Almost all markets have crashed, some slowly and some in a short period. The cause has been the implosion of money and credit, thanks to the investment made by banks in financial derivative instruments such as collateralised debt obligation (CDO), once described by Warren Buffet as "investment instruments of mass destruction". If one goes deeper to discover the cause of the current situation, it is the cheap money policy that created the technology and housing bubble along with the explosive rise in derivative instruments. It is amazing that no one among the watchdogs saw the problem associated with wildly imprudent lending to anyone, creditworthy or not. It is pure lunacy to lend to totally unworthy applicants by assigning finite risk when we know that the risk is close to infinite. They did it by creating sub-prime (lower than prime) mortgages with variable interest rates. So how do we come out of this economic turmoil?

First, I hope they are able to bring reasonable stability in both financial and housing markets by injecting the liquidity and lowering the interest rate. Though I am a strong believer in free markets, the current situation needs government participation to protect the taxpaying public. Government needs to take every possible step to keep unemployment under control, currently around 6 per cent, keeping below 7.5 per cent. As stated earlier, we need to focus on austerity and internal growth more so than the external. We need not increase the size of houses and automobiles that we use, but rather increase our Samskara to help ourselves and others in need. Samskara implies human impulses in sync with the nature. It is not desirable for an advanced economy to be dependent on imported energy. One way to reduce the dependence on petroleum is to wean ourselves away from the habit of driving big gas-consuming cars to smaller autos that would give close to 100 miles per gallon. It is true that wages are not on a par with productivity in Western countries, thanks to an abundant and cheap supply of labour in Asia. Another trend the world over, implemented by many governments, is not letting the economy fall into a deflationary cycle that could result in a depression that would create very high unemployment. Governments keep the cost of money low by keeping the interest rate low and injecting more money into the system. Maintaining a loose money policy helps governments manage large debt and employment.

In this economic environment, the losers are the creditors, retirees, and wage earners, and the winners are owners of hard assets and businesses with high growth. A large labour supply implies that there is a greater need for things requiring the mind and intellect in order to bring balance. Education, training, and Samskara help to balance each pair of opposites, and would enable wage earners to become more creative in competing to develop a demand for the products and services they provide.

Samskaric principles guide the training and culturing of physical impulses and reflexes, including the integration and development of harmony of pairs of opposites. Ruta is the Universal and Eternal Truth or Ultimate Reality or Brahman in its dynamic, temporal, material form. Ruta is Nature in its best mood, benevolent, loving, and truthful. It is the first evolute, the first incarnate of Nature. Samskara and Ruta are intimately related. Samskara is the energy and the feminine side of Ruta, which is operational through Samskara. When the somatic self is cultivated and develops Samskara, Ruta becomes accessible. Ruta is the spirit within the grain, the fragrance of the rose, and the joy in music. In short, Ruta is the essence of nature. God created Ruta, the first evolute of Nature — a very conceivable form of being, its second part being the finest form of intellect, and the source being the somatic self. Ruta is the force that creates rhythmic existence out of the anarchic disorder, harmony out of cacophony.

Table of Total Human Self Linked with Nature and Different Human Endeavour

Cosmic Energy	Matter, Earth	Space Avakash	Time Dependence
Genetics	Physical Body	Intuitive Mind	Intellect
DNA, Sperm	Organs: Brain, Heart	Love, Devotion	Reasoning
Seeds, Egg, Origin	Nerves, Senses, Reflexes	Belief, Intuition, Spontaneity	Logical, Self-Centered
Start, Initial Condition	Digest, Breath Actions, Walk	Revelation, Idealism	Control, Attention
News Media, Radio Talk	Executive Branch	Legislative Branch	Judiciary Branch
Stored Energy	Earth, Matter, Particles	Space, Continuous	Time
Information, Blueprint	Organisms, Organisations	Dream, Imagination	Dynamic Flow, Control
Noise, Chaos Information Start Initial State Roots	Numbers, Digits Arithmetic Many Quanta Branches	Analog, Geometry, Much, Waves, Fields, Fractal, Layered	Algebra, Calculus, (non) Linear, Diff. Equation, Programmes
Stored Action, Karma-Past Samskara	Action, Karma Yoga, Austerity, Training	Devotion, Bhakti Yoga, Love, Compassion, Fair Play	Knowledge Gyana Yoga, Attention, Control
Initial Capital Invest, Savings, Adam Smith	Goods/ Products, Services, Karl Marx	Vendors/ Suppliers, Manufacturer, Maynard Keynes	Consumer/Users, Demand, Milton Friedman
Originator Moses Divinity, Spirituality imbedded in Genes	Proletariat, Karl Marx Existent, Autonomous, Non-judgemental, Austerity	Love/Christ, Jung, Freud Sub-Rating, Transcendence, Immanence, Compassion	Law-giver, Kautilya, David Harmony, Complement, Control, Balance

6

Reviving the American Dream

ON March 11, 2011, when much of America was fast asleep, Japan was traumatized by a shock wave. A massive earthquake, as high as 9 on the Richter scale, shook the nation for over two minutes, causing unprecedented destruction in its wake. A powerful tsunami followed a few hours later, sharply deepening the gloom and destruction. It was the latest example of what can happen when a vast imbalance occurs in nature in the form of shifting tectonic plates underneath a country's surface.

Apparently something similar is at work in the global economic system, which is also now plagued by vast imbalances. They have already generated a violent storm in terms of what is now called The Great Recession that started in late 2007 and has lingered till this day in the form of 20 million jobless Americans. But since the imbalances have only worsened, we are now headed towards an economic earthquake that could be as disastrous as the tremor that hit Japan.

The previous chapters have described these imbalances in detail, and let me put them all together to see what concerted action can now be taken to ward off the coming disaster. They are as follows:

1. Huge budget deficits
2. Huge trade deficits or surpluses

3. Massive printing of money
4. An unprecedented oil price rise in a recession
5. Because of deregulation, banks enjoying vast profits with reduced lending
6. Income and wealth inequalities not seen in capitalism before
7. Vanishing manufacturing jobs

The rest of the chapter is an elaboration of these points and the required economic reforms.

Giant Budget Deficits

The whole world is now awash in giant budget deficits. Most economists attribute them to the popularity of Keynesian economics, but that is not accurate. Keynes never preached relentless deficits, which were needed in recessions and depressions to raise aggregate demand, but the deficits were to be matched with surplus budgets when boom came around. There would then be deficits and surpluses over the course of the business cycle, but not a debt accumulation. The U.S. debt pile, which was below a trillion in 1980, has grown into a mountain. The federal debt is now at $11 trillion, and it is rocketing at the rate of $1.5 trillion per year. In addition, almost all states, especially California and New York, have large deficits and debt. They either have to raise taxes or trim government spending or do both. And all this trimming is bound to be painful in terms of public employee layoffs and the elimination of services to which people are accustomed.

Conventional wisdom during the reign of President Bush junior was that homeowners could borrow nearly unlimited amounts of money without any consequences to the economy. The then Fed chairman Alan Greenspan saw no harm in generating borrowed prosperity. He was unaware that Nature dislikes imbalances, and somewhere things could go wrong unexpectedly to create misery for the borrowers, lenders and the economy. Things have not changed much even after Mr. Obama became president, because consumer borrowing was replaced by federal borrowing. Political wisdom since 2007 has been that the government can borrow unlimited quantities of money, stabilise the economy and face no undesired consequences. The Laws of Nature have been thwarted again, and this is simply ominous.

The United States indeed has been able to borrow trillions from abroad, because it is a military superpower, a consuming powerhouse and a key-currency nation. So far its borrowing has not had a bad effect on its financial institutions, although, as argued later, this practice has decimated its manufacturing and lowered real wages for millions of workers. Foreign countries simply accept paper dollars or American government bonds for their surplus goods exported to the United States. But what about other nations, which have also been accumulating debt at lofty rates to fight unemployment and reward government employees with generous pensions and healthcare benefits? Some Euro-zone nations have been as reckless as the United States in their foreign borrowing. Greece, Spain, Portugal and Ireland, among others, have borrowed trillions as if there is no tomorrow. But since 2009 they have faced the so-called "sovereign debt" crisis. Their lenders are not sure if they will get their money back in entirety. So such nations face sharply higher interest rates, which have slowed their economies.

The sovereign debt crisis emerged in full swing in mid 2010, when Greece was on the verge of defaulting on its foreign debt. Greek budget deficit had turned out to be larger than expected and it was not clear if the nation could service its giant debt. The previous chapter talked about the clustering property of nature. The property simply means that upward or downward trends occur for a while because events occur in a cluster. Otherwise there would be no discernible trends, but only random fluctuations, because a number of events with similar effects have to occur before a trend is formed. In any case, when Greece appeared to be on the verge of default, many other nations also appeared to be in the same boat. They included Portugal, Spain, Ireland, Poland, Hungary and even Russia. This illustrates how events tend to occur in clusters. As the saying goes, when it rains it pours.

Needless to say, the Euro-zone was shaken, and many even predicted the demise of the euro, which sank sharply from around 1.4 to the dollar to about 1.1. Many European banks had loaned large sums to Greek government and they were in danger of losing a lot of money. Naturally, the rest of Europe had to do something, rather than let the banks suffer the consequences of their reckless lending. Once again there was a bailout, this time of Greece and of other potential defaulters. Euro-zone governments such as Germany and France created a trillion euro fund that would lend money to governments in danger of default and buy their bonds at low interest rates. This is how global financial markets calmed down, and oil and share markets resumed their task of speculation.

Something similar could happen to the United States, which has been already stripped by Standard & Poor of its AAA debt rating. If the dollar loses its appeal abroad, our interest rates could jump and reignite the flames of recession. We may not be able to see why and when this would happen, but the Euro-zone debtors also did not foresee any problems regarding their foreign debts. The point is that when imbalances occur and natural laws are violated, some Black Swan event occurs and destroys the house of cards. People are then caught off-guard and lament their earlier recklessness, but by then it is too late. So the moral is that we should start reducing government spending and the budget deficit until it is eliminated in the future. Fortunately, thanks to the Tea Party movement, politicians are now beginning to heed to the debt pile. Hopefully, they will do something serious about it.

However, there are some economists who think that the U.S. budget deficit should rise even above the $1.5 trillion mark to reduce unemployment. Noble laureate Paul Krugman of Princeton University is the chief proponent of this view. He argues that this is the only way to trim joblessness below the 20 million level that has prevailed since 2008. On paper the argument is valid, because if the government cuts its deficit, output could fall and unemployment could go up. But the recent experience from the sovereign-debt crisis suggests that unlimited budget deficits have their costs in terms of higher interest rates and potentially bigger problems. Japan's experience since 1990 also points to the same thing, namely postponing genuine reforms by relentlessly increasing government spending is no sure way to prosperity. In fact, the opposite can happen. Japan has been stagnant for over two decades in spite of its debt pile, with no decline in unemployment.

The federal deficit no longer generates the return it did in the 1960s. At that time a 1 per cent deficit was associated with annual GDP growth of 4.5 per cent. From Bush-Cheney to Obama-Biden, the deficit has exceeded 10 per cent of GDP, yet growth has averaged below 3 per cent. Clearly, deficits are not the panacea they used to be in the past.

Trade Deficits and Surpluses

The other major imbalance in the world is that few nations have balanced trade. Some such as the United States and Australia have large deficits and other, such as China, the Asian tigers and Germany, have large surpluses in their foreign accounts. As explained in chapter 4, when the gap between labour productivity and the real wage increases, supply exceeds demand and then the country keeps its currency artificially low to generate a trade surplus to fill the supply-demand gap and keep its factories running. It keeps its employment high but only by exporting unemployment to trade-deficit nations. The United States also has a large wage-productivity gap, but it has encouraged so much consumer borrowing that its demand has consistently run ahead of its supply, and this excess demand is its trade deficit. Another reason for the high U.S. deficit is international financial deregulation, which is explained below in the section on deregulation.

American trade deficit also stems from the fact that cheap imports from abroad have all but destroyed the U.S. manufacturing base. The nation just does not produce the variety of goods that it did during the 1950s and the 1960s. So there is not much the country can export. Limited manufacturing also means a limited living standard, because the manufacturing wage normally exceeds the average wage in service industries that employ over 75 per cent of the U.S. workforce. This is because in manufacturing a nation builds products, whereas in services those products are repaired. And the repair work is far less valuable then the production work.

The havoc caused by American trade debacle on manufacturing cannot be exaggerated. According to the *Economic Report of the President*, some 11.5 million people out of a labour force of 150 million worked in manufacturing in 2010. This turns out to be less than 8 per cent. Now compare this to the situation in 1800 when the nation was primarily an agrarian economy. At that time about 6 per cent of the workforce was employed in manufacturing. How far are we from that state now? Not much. The United States is essentially back to the beginning of its industrial revolution, as far as manufacturing is concerned. Not surprisingly, the nation's living standard is also moving back towards the pre-industrialization days.

It is one thing to have free trade, and totally another to have a deficit-ridden trade. Early proponents and founders of the free trade doctrine did not envision giant trade deficits. They believed in balanced trade, which was produced by the gold standard. A deficit nation had to pay for excess imports with gold; this trimmed its money supply, which was also linked to its gold stockpile. The fall in money supply lowered its prices, and in turn stimulated exports, until the trade was in balance. Today everything is topsy-turvy. Money supply is no longer linked to gold or anything else; nations are happy to accept dollars for their surplus production. There is no compulsion for disciplined economic policies. So, imbalances keep growing.

In order to revive manufacturing, trade surplus nations must be compelled to follow free trade just as the United States and Europe do. Currency manipulation violates free commerce. The Asian tigers and China are the main manipulators. They should be so declared, and then under the WTO rules that prohibit subsidies the United States will be able to impose trade restrictions on such nations. That will then quickly revive American manufacturing, create high-paying jobs and trim unemployment.

Gottfried Haberler, a Harvard economist, proved in 1950 that tariffs raise the nation's living standard when there is large-scale unemployment. This economist was generally in favour of free trade, except in the presence of high joblessness, which is what plagues the U.S. and European economies today. So deficit-ridden free trade must be abandoned until unemployment is eradicated.

Printing of Money

Another irresponsible policy today is the uncontrolled money-printing by the world's central banks. Fed chairman Ben Bernanke likes to say that he is not printing money, but just buying Treasury debt in bond markets. Any time the Fed buys anything from the private sector, it creates money, either by printing it or by writing a check for the purchase, because the check is eventually deposited in a bank, which then has more money. There is no transparency in what central banks are doing around the globe. But it is common knowledge that trillions have been printed or created to bailout several banks that had offered cheap, no-downpayment loans to homeowners in the past, thereby generating a housing bubble all over the planet. The banks and their employees reaped large fees and bonuses, but then their loans soured and generated a housing and banking crisis, and a serious recession.

The Fed is not worried about inflation, and in justification it points to the muted rise in the consumer price index (CPI) since 2007. However, the CPI is not the only gauge of soaring prices. There are two types of inflation — commodity inflation of the CPI, and asset inflation. Both produce worrisome consequences. Asset inflation, whereby prices soar for shares, oil and gold, is just as bad as the rise in the cost of living. The doubling of the gold price between 2007 and 2011 shows that the public is worried about the CPI inflation as well as the excessive printing of money. Share prices also rocketed from March 2009 to early 2011 as if the United States was in the midst of a boom. Even though GDP growth averaged less than 3 per cent, and joblessness remained steady at 20 million, the Dow soared 90 per cent in just two years. Something that goes up sharply also comes down sharply, and when it falls, it really hurts and sours the economy. So asset inflation can be really harmful, and when money supply soars to generate it, the policy is wrong and the end result can be very painful. Ask Alan Greenspan, who presided over stock market bubbles and their crashes in 2000 and then in 2008. There are no free markets, more so after the 2008-2009 market crash. Markets are manipulated by institutions, often with the blessing of the government, for political and economic advantage.

Perhaps the worst consequences of asset inflation have been felt in the oil market. In my memory, this is the first recession, where the price of oil has not really declined. During the economic stagnation of the 1980s, the international price fell below $10 per barrel. The recession of 1979-1982 was long gone, but a stagnant economy saw oil drop sharply in 1986. The same thing happened during the short recession of 1990 and the Asian Flu recession of 1998-1999. The reason why oil sinks in a slump is that while the industrial demand for the product falls strongly, its production does not. So the price plummets.

This time around, however, the recession is the worst since the 1930s, yet oil went as high as $147 per barrel in 2008, and remained around $80 during much of 2009 and 2010, although at one point during 2008, it dropped to as low as $32. It should be clear that supply and demand after March 2009. Indeed institutions and funds made a lot of money, but expensive oil creates job losses and delays a good recovery. The point of it all is that there are other costs to excessive money creation, which Bernanke has not recognised.

There is also hidden inflation that many have not noticed. The cost of essential goods and services has risen much faster than the CPI. But share markets and the Fed focus on the so-called core CPI that excludes food and energy. The bar chart from Casey Research shows that the annual price of wheat, oats, pork and cotton has gone up 60 per cent, while the price of canola, sugar, copper, heating oil, gasoline, coffee and beef has surged over 20 per cent.

All this points to a need for monetary discipline. What then should be the annual growth in money supply? Milton Friedman gives us the answer. He used the classical economists' quantity theory of money to offer a monetarist rule. The theory relies upon the well-known exchange equation:

$$MV = PY$$

Here M is money supply, V, the velocity of money in circulation, P is the average price such as the CPI, and Y is real GDP. Friedman believes that normally V remains constant as it depends on bank lending and how much money people want to keep as cash in their wallets. If P is to be kept constant, i.e. if the inflation rate is to be zero, then M should grow at the same rate as Y or the GDP. It can be shown from the equation that if P and V are constant, then

Money growth = GDP growth

which is about 4 per cent per year over the long run. Hence annual money creation, according to Friedman, should not exceed this figure. But money growth has far exceeded this rule, and that is why there has been asset inflation as well as a strong surge of food and energy prices.

Another type of money growth rule is offered by the proponents of gold and silver standard, where money supply is linked to the nation's stock of gold and silver. Since this stock does not grow fast, money growth is also restrained. In addition, the gold and silver standard, as argued above, does not permit unlimited trade deficits. This is then another argument in its favour, and I believe reversion to this standard will go a long way in restoring price stability and the revival of U.S. manufacturing.

Historically, gold standard provided a stable debt to GDP ratio of about 1.6. This ratio started to rise uncontrollably after 1971 when the gold standard was removed, and currently (End of 2010) it is about 3.6. Anchoring currency (think of it as blood flowing in the economic body) to gold and/or silver regulates the currency flow, and provides nutrition efficiently to the economic body. Unanchored fiat currency flow often accelerates to the level of uncontrolled velocity creating the economic boom and bust. This is what happened in the late

1970s in the United States. Similarly, hyperinflations of the past, such as those in Germany (1920s) and Brazil (1980s and 1990s), occurred because of a sharp rise in the velocity of money, so much so that people tried to spend money the moment they received any cash, fearing that their cash could lose value the next day, or even the next hour. But anchoring currency to gold and silver would remove the threat of such high inflation.

Deregulation

Regulations don't matter anymore in the determination of the oil price, which now moves violently and most unexpectedly. Otherwise, with the globe suffering the terrible recession, the price should have dropped to $10, at least for a few months, as it used to do in the past.

The main reason for the failure of the laws of supply and demand in oil is huge speculation along with a much larger money supply, which has been fostered by all that money that the banks have received from their bailouts. The banks are unwilling to lend much in a weak economy, but with so much cash piling up in the vaults of financial institutions they, along with hedge funds, are busy using it in speculation, especially in oil, gold and copper. The prices of such assets soared once the stock market recovered.

Ever since 1981 many industries have been deregulated, some with positive results and some with negative consequences. When this policy encourages competition among firms, the effects are positive, but when it stimulates speculation, the impact is mostly negative. Thus, deregulation of airlines and telecommunications done in the early 1980s increased competition in these areas; as a result airline fares fell sharply, and so did phone charges. I remember the days when I had to pay $2 per minute to speak to my family in India, but now I can do this for less than a quarter. I also remember when I used to cringe while flying from Los Angeles to New York. The economy class air fare ran into thousands, at least in terms of today's prices. Now you can fly the same route for as low as $500. This type of deregulation has had a strongly positive effect for the consumer.

However, deregulation was also extended in the 1990s to the financial sector, especially with the repeal of the Glass-Steagall Act (GSA), which had barred commercial banks to conduct investment banking activities. Until the Act's repeal the banks were not allowed to deal with stocks and their derivatives, but now they were able to do what they had done during the 1920s, i.e. delve in stocks and then create a stock market bubble, with disastrous consequences in the 1930s. This time too, bubbles dutifully followed the financial deregulation, only to climax into crashes. The point is that industrial deregulation is good, but financial deregulation, particularly when products developed by Wall Street are totally opaque, is bad for the economy.

There were also some unintended consequences of the GSA's repeal. It led to international financial deregulation as well. Until 1995, when the WTO (World Trade Organization) displaced the GATT (The General Agreement on Tariffs and Trade of 1944), individuals in many countries such as Japan were not permitted to transfer money abroad. The financial institutions could do that, but not individuals. International finance's deregulation changed it all, with unexpected effects on America's foreign commerce, because the dollar could not fall in spite of the rising trade deficit. Such was not the case during the 1970s and the 1980s, when a nation's trade deficit would routinely result in currency depreciation, which in turn eliminated the deficit. This, however, is no longer true.

Once international finance was deregulated, individuals and institutions in trade-surplus nations increasingly invested their dollars into U.S. government bonds and other assets.

Countries like China, Japan, Korea and Saudi Arabia purchased these bonds in great quantities, thereby preventing the needed fall in the dollar. So the trade deficit could not correct itself, and kept rising with no end in sight. The deficit in turn decimated U.S. manufacturing. Thus, financial deregulation, domestic and international, had deleterious, though unintended, consequences.

There is a fundamental reason why banks should not be allowed to dabble in risky ventures. If they were dealing with their own money, they would not be so fearless, but they are dealing with other people's money (OPEOM), which we know is quite addictive. When they are reasonably certain that they will be bailed out in case of major losses, they tend to be reckless in speculation, and when their bets misfire they can cause havoc in the economy. The world learnt this lesson painfully during the Great Depression and the United States enacted the GSA in the 1930s, but in 1999 this was all forgotten as the GSA was repealed that year. Why we repeat our mistakes is unfathomable. The biggest problem deregulation has created is the ballooning of a very opaque derivative market. The notional value today (March 2011) of the derivative market is over 700 trillion dollars, about ten times the total world GDP of about 65 trillion dollars (2009). The problem associated with the elephant-sized derivative market has also been described as financial instruments of mass destruction.

America should put an end to financial deregulation, but deregulation of industries should be given top priority, especially in energy. The reason why oil topped $147 per barrel in 2008 is that in addition to speculation there are now two oil cartels, one international and the other domestic. The international cartel is, of course, the OPEC, or the Organisation of Petroleum Exporting Countries, but there is also a domestic cartel that includes the so-called five sisters — Exxon-Mobile, Texaco-Chevron, Royal Dutch Shell, British Petroleum and Conoco-Phillips.

Some of these names suggest that they were formed from mergers of large companies such as Exxon and Mobil. In fact, there were more than 2,600 mergers in the oil industry in the 1990s. Mergers among large companies are what generate cartels. When competition declines, prices generally rise. It is not surprising, therefore, that two cartels, instead of one, would create extremely high prices. If deregulation were to occur in domestic oil, and some of the firms were broken up to increase competition, the way AT&T was broken in 1983, then just like phone charges, the oil price will fall. In fact, no new laws need be passed; only the existing anti-trust laws should be enforced. The United States can follow its own precedent in the way Standard Oil was broken up into 16 independent companies in 1911, only to be followed by a visible decline in the price of gasoline. The size of a corporation matters. I believe there should not be any institution that has become "Too Big to Fail".

Income and Wealth Disparity

The biggest problem in the world today is rocketing inequality in income and wealth. Conventional economists usually shun this subject, just as they did in the 1920s, but now the inequality is the highest in the history of capitalism and cannot be ignored anymore. Barely 1 per cent of families own more than 40 per cent of wealth in the United States; the bottom 20 per cent have just 3 per cent share of income. Not only does this disparity have social consequences in terms of crime and divorce rates, as the low-income family simply finds it hard to cope with day-today pressures of life, it also has very harsh economic consequences. Professors Raghuram Rajan and Ravi Batra have argued that consumer debt problems arose because of growing inequality in the 1990s and 2000s. They both were critical of Greenspan who ignored this development and fostered a culture of reckless indebtedness. As wages stagnated and Greenspan brought interest rates down to fight the onslaught of share price crashes, consumers and homeowners increasingly borrowed money in a desperate attempt to maintain their lifestyles. The end result was a credit binge, a housing boom and eventual housing collapse. But because of stagnant wages, profits went sky-high, and so did executive compensation and income and wealth disparities.

Some of the reforms I have suggested above will also reduce inequality. For instance, balancing our trade by compelling trade-surplus nations to follow free trade and revalue their currencies will revive U.S. manufacturing and create high paying jobs. As the middle class salaries go up, inequality would fall. Similarly, restraining money growth will reduce inflation and the cost of living, which in turn will raise the purchasing power of people's savings as well as their incomes. Repealing financial deregulation will induce banks to pay attention to their real purpose, which is to lend money to needy businesses. This will stimulate investment as well as employment and the economy. When banks no longer are able to make money from financial derivatives, they will have to find other ways to make a profit; so they will have an incentive to give loans and thus lubricate the economy.

Oil speculation will fall if banks are not permitted to use people's deposits for non-lending activities. This will also help the middle class. Thus, the reforms suggested above will tend to mitigate income and wealth disparities.

Clustering of Events and Conclusion

I have repeatedly referred to clustering of events, because it is very important to see how nature works and how we should not be complacent in the wake of growing imbalances. This property of nature suggests that first, we should not allow imbalances to emerge at all, and second, if they have emerged, we should not wait till a calamity arises and brings misery for a long time.

From March 9, 2009 to February 18, 2011, there was a relentless rise in share prices, spawning yet another bubble, which was nothing new as such events have been occurring with regularity in the United States and the rest of the world. There were stock market bubbles in the 1980s, then in the 1990s, and then again between 2004 and 2007. They had all crashed, but major investors had been bailed out. However, the latest bubble was even more explosive than any seen before. The Dow Jones Index (Dow) nearly doubled in less than two years, from about 6700 to over 12,400. Was the economy booming, or unemployment sinking? No. That is what separates this bubble from all others. It happened in an environment of less than 3 per cent GDP growth, even as layoffs continued. It happened even as General Motors and Chrysler declared bankruptcy and had to be bailed out. It occurred even as oil resumed its upward march and jumped from a low of $32 per barrel to around $80. However, share markets ignored all these negative factors and kept rising.

Between December 2010 and February 2011, the Dow rose for 8 straight weeks. Investors were giddy with hefty profits. But then came a cluster of events that even blindly speculating bankers and hedge funds could not ignore. The Mid-East was in turmoil, not from the regular Palestinian-Israeli conflict, but because the poor and oppressed masses were up in revolt against corrupt dictators and their cronies. First, Tunisia was in revolt, then Egypt. In January and February, the presidents of both countries were overthrown, followed by a civil war in Libya. Furthermore, the flame of freedom spread like a wildfire, as dictators in Yemen, Algeria, Oman, Bahrain, and even Saudi Arabia faced protests from their once docile masses. The rest of the world could not but notice the sudden burst of revolutions. Oil speculators now had a field day. Libya's oil production was shut down, and even though this reduced global supply by only 2 per cent, oil price jumped by more than 20 per cent in just two weeks. Even the diehard speculators could not ignore this jump, and share prices started to retreat. The Dow and S&P 500 peaked on February 18, 2011 for this cycle.

Initially, the retreat was tolerable and appeared to be short-lived. But the unprecedented earthquake of Japan changed that picture. First there was the terrible earthquake, then a powerful tsunami, followed by fires in four nuclear reactors, creating the possibility of nuclear meltdown. This was too much, and in just a month the Dow was down 8 per cent. This is where things stood at the time of this writing. Notice the cluster of problems for share markets. First the soaring oil, then a huge loss in Japan, with the third largest economy in the world. It appears that the latest bubble will also burst like all others before, and then the economy will be even worse.

What do we learn from these historical events? In sum, not much has changed in terms of economic policy from Bush-Cheney to Obama-Biden. The deficit went up, but few jobs were created; recession ended in terms of GDP decline, as GDP growth became positive, but 20 million people still remained out of work. The stock market did recover strongly, thereby creating an impression of a healthy economy; but this was another bubble, and perhaps the worst in history in the sense it occurred in the backdrop of a fragile economy.

Money creation remained as hefty as before. In fact, on top of quantitative-easing (QE) of 2008 and 2009, in 2010 Mr. Bernanke introduced QE2, which pumped another dose of monetary stimulus into the economy. Mercifully, this was only worth $600 billion, not the two or three trillion that many believe the Fed had injected into the banking system under QE1. What will the Fed do when there is another crash, which is inevitable, because every bubble bursts eventually?

It is clear that we need to reduce the federal deficit, restrain money growth, enforce anti-trust laws, end financial deregulation, perhaps even return to the gold standard, and, above all, eliminate the trade deficit by declaring China and other trade surplus areas as currency manipulators. When such reforms are introduced, global imbalances will decline, and economic policy will conform to the infallible laws of nature. U.S. manufacturing base will revive. Prosperity will then return and the living standard will rise for all, not just for the wealthy few.

I would also like to see more balance and harmony between the opposites of a pair that would ultimately complement each other. More needs to be done to avoid polarisation and build bridges between feuding opposites. The modern world is dominated by a Western world view, as a result of the old colonial mindset. But the legacy of the East has always been the power of knowledge. For a solution to inequalities, a clear perception of the problems is first necessary. It seems every pair, liberals and conservatives, labour and management, paper currencies and inflation hedges, and many more . . . all seem to be out of balance. Then there are problems of corruption at the highest levels in India and GAPONOMICS, implying a widening gap between the rich and the poor in Western countries, featured in the March 12th 2011 issue of *The Economist* magazine. What we need is life-education, not merely professional education without morality, which has led us to the exploitative world of today. We need education of the heart. I hope greater emphasis is put on such education at every level. Education that unifies humanity, but maintains individual autonomy, that stimulates the highest level of creativity, should become our universal currency, the currency of the mind, together with the currency anchored to an acceptable standard such as gold and silver needed for a sound economy and a healthy body — with hopefully very positive results.

Appendix A
Aphorisms Applied to Economics

- Organisms and organisations (O&O) must learn to find their multi-dimensional space and boundaries, unique to each of them, and learn to live close to the centre. If one hits a boundary, one could perish. Boundaries are not fine lines of demarcation but a cluster of barriers with rising heights, occupying a portion of the living space.
- O&O are autonomous, self-organising, and ceaselessly exchange matter and energy with Nature. Nature and O&O co-exist and are symbiotic. Knowledge of Nature helps man to discover the solution of human existential problems. However, Nature will never be a slave of man.
- Hindsight is always 20/20; however, Nature is 80/20. Events occur in clusters, things form clusters, and are almost never evenly distributed. Often the change occurs in jumps; when it rains, it pours. Examples of clusters are — blood clots, stars, automobiles on the freeway, people of the same cultural background. Prices of goods, services, and stocks cluster around the mean in time domain.
- Among few supreme laws of Nature, the law of demand and supply, discovered by Adam Smith, is one of them. Demand, supply, and price seem to be

analogous to voltage, current, and resistance of Ohm's Law in electricity.

- Adversity promotes solidarity among most O&O, if not all, and affluence retards and often reverses the process of solidarity. This is one of the causes, among many, that create economic cycles.
- Four basic units of the total human self consisting of two pairs of opposites, and symbiotic with Nature are genetics, the physical body, the intuitive mind, and the intellectual mind; just as length, mass, time, ampere, and lumen are the basic units of measurement in physics. Components of every field of human endeavour can be associated with these four basic units of the total human self.
- In the political and economic domain, genetics is associated with the news media, savings as initial capital, and GDP; physical body is associated with executive branch, employment and the goods and services produced; intuitive mind is associated with the legislative branch, the rate of inflation and the productivity; and the intellectual mind is associated with the judiciary, the interest rate, and the consumption.
- Autonomy of order at every level and layer, probably prolongs the life of the order. Autonomy implies minimum external interaction. Autonomy slows down the process of decay. An order that adapts to its environment also extends its life. The mixing of orders may accelerate the decay. The implication is that organisations should function giving maximum autonomy at every level.
- Free will and freedom to choose is a gift from Nature to humanity. However, this gift is relative in value. It

cannot be absolute since Nature assures and guarantees the availability of an opposite to every dimension, even in matters of free will and the freedom to choose. (matters of globalisation)

- Creative order-generating activity of the human mind is at least as significant as if not more than the natural evolutionary processes, that give birth to the human body — mother of the human mind.
- The outcomes of cultural evolution generated by organisms are less complex and less diverse than those generated by biological evolution. Cultural evolution is visible, knowable and occurs in a much shorter time span than invisible biological evolution.
- Biological evolution of human body is natural, unpredictable, and not accessible to the human mind. Cultural evolution and revolution is associated with the human mind and is predictable; tools such as mathematics, language, and computers are employed for the purpose.
- Organisms, organisations, and markets evolve. Evolution implies long periods of equilibrium, or, a very slow change with short periods of quantum change, with increasing complexity.
- Economy is about scarce resources (e.g. money) having many uses (ways to spend it). It is also about finding the right allocation of these resources for different needs.
- A free market economic system, along with appropriate checks and balances, is probably the most natural compared to others, such as communism. However, it will keep changing, evolving, and adapting to its environment.

- Economy grows on capital formation where capital includes roads, buildings, machines, money, and trained manpower; consumption does not provide the growth of capital.
- Gresham's Law, often stated as "bad money drives out good money", also implies that money goes where it is treated the best. The law seems to apply in politics also, bad politicians drive out good ones (e.g. India).
- Gold (silver), based upon human experience of many millennia, is money and holds its purchasing power constant forever. It becomes an asset of choice when real interest rates are negative. However, there is an inverse relationship between the price of gold and the prevailing real interest rate.
- The price of gold is also the reciprocal of the faith and the trust reposed in institutions of managed currencies.
- Deflation occurs in two ways; the bad deflation occurs in a declining economy due to the over-extended debt that causes businesses to fail and price declines. A good deflation occurs in a growing economy and increased productivity, causing prices to decline.
- There is always some good in the worst of us and some bad in the best of us. It is not meant for us to judge others. A "holier than thou" attitude creates more problems than solutions. It also implies that one should not throw the baby with the bath water.
- Within one's domain, one should be inclusive of others. The process of transcendence towards higher levels is unidirectional. Regression should be avoided though there are exceptions.
- Autonomy is the prerequisite to detachment. Detachment is the prerequisite to sub-ration, and sub-ration is the prerequisite to transcendence. The total

human self needs to experience both transcendence and immanence. Creative destruction is an example of detachment and sub-ration. We sub-rated and detached from the horse and buggy and replaced them with automobiles.

- There is, in an idealised God's nature, an infinite quantity of information. However, the information accessible to human mind is only that information that can come across and be observed by the equipment given to man (Anthropic Principle). Man chooses what, why, and how to observe and interpret results.
- One needs to put more emphasis on the positive and not the negative. The ancient sages believed the greed of anything, including knowledge, is as harmful as the greed of gold. Greed implies attachment, hindering detachment. (Refer to market psychology.)
- Expansion and clustering are common in Nature and in the human psyche. Astronomers accept galactic expansions as real; empires and corporations tend to expand. Our knowledge of Nature is expanding, even exploding, thanks to the external cultural evolution that includes high-tech homes, automobiles, telephones, computers, and the Internet.
- Earth is not only a living organism but is also self-aware, through all her living creatures, organisations, and financial markets. There are constant battles between these forces for the well-being of mother earth just as there are ongoing battles of cells within the human body, to survive and prosper.
- Spontaneous creativity happens only when every human faculty or every constituent component of an organisation complements each of the others and works in harmony. An idealistic and creative human

mind is a bigger monument of Nature than a temple or a cathedral. (Best ways to solve problems, conclusion.)

- There is a quantum analog of the total human self, which exists as a self-centred individual that can transcend to a selfless non-local universal consciousness, just as a sub-atomic particle like an electron can transform from an individual particle to an ever-expanding and unifying wave. Therefore, becoming selfless has to be the ultimate goal in the life of every human being.
- There is no absolute determinism in a chaotic universe. One need not brood over the dead past, nor worry about the unborn future, but must act in the living present. Stated differently: Yesterday is history, tomorrow is mystery, and today is a gift; that is why it is called "the present".

Appendix B
Market Psychology / Market Cliches

The behaviours of crowds and individuals as well as organisations follow the laws of Nature. A crowd's behaviour can, at first glance, seem chaotic, directionless, and without focus — somewhat like our own minds with random thoughts. Yet, just as a hurricane close-up may appear to be a torrent of wind and rain, a satellite view from above shows it to be a circling mass of air and water following specific natural laws. It has a central "eye," rising and falling barometric zones, and a path that is determined by the warm and cold currents of water and air that created it. Human existence may seem directionless and chaotic, but time eventually reveals a "method to its madness." Markets of stocks, bonds and commodities similarly move to natural laws. They appear to mimic the directionless mass psychology of crowds, and follow certain laws that move them through intervals of "bulls" and "bears," which seen from "above" have a logical pattern and even a natural order.

The laws of evolution and of demand and supply are applicable to every level of human existence, including the rising and falling of markets. Markets are influenced by what wages are paid to workers; what workers pay for food, rent or mortgage; and where they travel. The pricing pattern of stocks in the short duration may resemble the erratic movement of fish in water, or perhaps the pattern of a chaotic electronic signal of an amplifier with no input signal. But with some insight and a new perspective on a stock, it may reveal a definite long-term pattern. Markets are always evolving but often chaotic. The regulatory agencies tend to devise laws so that the catastrophic fluctuations and volatility of the market are minimised. However, neither Nature nor the market can be tamed by man for ever.

Markets, like Nature, are fractal, implying that they have self-similar patterns. The price-chart patterns of Dow Jones Industrial are similar, regardless of the time coordinate, which could be in units of hours, days, weeks or months. The tree is an example in Nature, where the smallest branch resembles the largest. Another example is that of a seashore line—the patterns are self-similar, no matter from what height one observes the shoreline.

Market setbacks often seem to bring "death" to the market as it happened in 1987, 2000, 2002, and 2008. However with time, the market becomes "alive" again and functions as anticipated. It is amazing how the market has a capacity to become organised out of a chaotic situation. It seems to have the same attitude as many organisations made of various individuals with their own ideas, which eventually come together to create a cohesive whole. Sometimes, chaos just needs time to come together. Orders of the world are created out of chaos. So too we see this with markets and organisations. We have observed how time heals almost all wounds, physical as well as mental. Destructive orders like tsunamis cause deep wounds or even death; creative orders support progress.

Let us consider some market cliches based on the laws of Nature:

1. What goes up comes down. This refers to the law of gravity and the law of demand and supply. If, for example, demand goes up for a product that just came on the market and the supply is not enough, the price

of the product goes up. However as supply catches up with demand, which usually happens because suppliers will produce more to make more profits, then the price of a particular product stabilises. In time, an "over-supply" will make the price go down.

2. There is absolutely no free lunch, not now or ever! Though some advertisements say that you get something for nothing, this is not true. One always gives something that is valuable to the advertiser. This is analogous to the laws of conservation of mass and energy. Mass or energy cannot be destroyed without accounting for it.
3. Growth engines run our economy. Often we hear that a particular sector — for example, information technology — is the "growth engine" of today's economy. Is there an engine in economy? The answer is actually "yes," because the economy can stall, accelerate or even overheat. Economies can even be "jump-started." So, yes, the economy has many engines to make it move.
4. Markets gyrate between greed and fear, the two extremes of mass psychology. They are among the pairs of opposites discussed in Chapter 5. Our ancestors feared Nature due to ignorance of it. Ignorance is also the cause of fear and greed. Markets get oversold since fear overrules reason, causing indiscriminate selling creating investment opportunities. Greed causes markets to be overbought creating trap to loose money. Another similar cliche of the market is to buy low and sell high. Get in early at the ground level and get out when the price has gone to the stratosphere. But momentum players say, "Buy high and sell higher."

5. Hindsight is always 20/20, but markets, like Nature, are 80/20.
6. One should not fight the Tape or the Fed. One should never go against the markets. Trend is your friend until it ends — ride the "waves" of the price movement. The trend is on track even if it is flat. Watch the slope and get off the slope if it drops like a rock. Do not stay too long if the trend becomes a tsunami. Do not ever think you have power over the waves. Get rid of arrogance and be humble to the market. Neither the market nor Nature is anyone's slave. One needs to remove the deadly foursome — hope, greed, vanity, and fear — to become a successful player.
7. Life is a game — so is playing the market. Contrary to what Einstein believed, God does play dice and God doesn't play favourites. Investors need to be emotionally detached but enjoy the ride of the market when it is climbing the wall of worries.
8. Money flows where it receives the best treatment. Money flows where it finds the best return with minimum risks. A superior return creates a force of attraction similar to a gravitational force. Money or capital is liquid and it flows whenever there is force or pressure applied to it. Capital, like power, is feminine, as was discussed in detail in Chapter 3. The feminine Goddess Lakshmi in Indian tradition is the provider of wealth and material well-being.
9. Statistically, Monday is the worst day of the week for selling. Recall that most heart attacks occur on Monday, due to mental conditioning.
10. The market resembles a pod of peas. The market is a Place where the Power to Pick and Purchase stocks will Produce Profits for Patient People. In the "pod of

peas," one needs to consider companies providing indispensable goods with increasing profits.

11. No two bull markets are alike, since they are orders of different attributes. All bear markets resemble death and are similar to chaos.
12. There is no such thing as an absolutely safe investment, since Nature does not allow anything absolute and unchanging. We know that relativity rules in Nature and certainly it rules in the market. The high interest rates of over 15 per cent were harmful to the U.S. economy in the 1980s; however, less than half of that rate busted the tech bubble in 2000.
13. The randomness of stock prices is comparable or similar to the random motion of air molecules.
14. The greater the randomness of the stock prices, the higher or lower the stock price could move and therefore, the higher the premium (cost) of the stock options (puts and calls).
15. The high frequency trading is likely to become more common as stock exchanges get closer and closer to an automated system.
16. Trading frequency increases based upon relevant news. For example, more traders will buy the stock of an oil company after the announcement of a large oil discovery.
17. "All this works great, until is does not." Everything falls apart when a "Black Swan" event takes place, i.e. an event like a tsunami that exists at the farthest reaches of probability.
18. Attributes of "Black Swan" events include that it is unpredictable, it is an extremely rare event, and it is unquantifiable. It carries a massive impact wherever

and whenever it occurs. Furthermore, after the event occurs and becomes history, scholars tend to make it predictable, i.e. scholars tend to bring it within the probability distribution curve, i.e. they tend to make a natural 80/20 "Black Swan" event into a 20/20 "White Swan" event.

19. A computer algorithm for stock trading is good until it fails to generate a profit. And in time, the lifespan of a trading algorithm will shorten and shorten.
20. Today, all markets are interconnected. Complexities of derivatives have linked markets together that would not normally be linked. A rise or drop in equity markets could cause the same effect in commodity markets. The correlation coefficient of one market with respect to another is never constant.
21. The knowledge of economics is imperfect and will remain imperfect since Nature and human psychology will resist perfection.

Increasing successful tighter controls over markets should increase the agility and decrease fluctuations of the price movement. This is analogous to brain waves (EEG); an alert brain implies tighter control or having waves of higher frequencies and lower amplitude and vice versa.

There is interdependence between markets and other phenomena. For example, every dynamic system in Nature exchanges matter and energy to survive. Living organisms need food, water and an air supply to exist and are self-organising, meaning they choose their structure and function.

Markets function like living organisms. Just as blood in our systems nourishes all our cells and provides oxygen and energy, currency provides sustenance to the market and an economy. Excessive currency in circulation will create inflation, similar to excess blood in an obese human body. In an electrical system, voltage causes the current flow, similar to blood pressure, which causes the flow of blood. Likewise in an economy, the supply of goods and services is a type of "current" with "demand" being equivalent to electrical voltage — pumps, engines, batteries and demand are needed to create the flow. In a market economy, the price of goods is a form of resistance or regulator of the flow — a higher price causes less demand. Diversification of investment can help minimise risk, the same as eating diverse foods helps to maintain good health.

With a heart free of hatred, a mind free of worries and anxieties, live simply, love generously without conditions, give more, expect less, care deeply, speak kindly, and play the game of life without fear. We are players and the world is a stage — there is a moment to enter the stage, and a moment to depart. Stay active and involved. Participate without attachment. Remain nimble and agile. Then the game of life becomes rewarding.

Appendix C
Free Market Quotes

I deny the power of the government to making paper money, or anything else a legal tender. — Thomas Jefferson

I place [the] economy among the first and most important virtues, and public debt as the greatest of dangers to be feared . . . we must not let our rulers load us with perpetual debt. We must make our choice between economy and liberty . . . or profusion and servitude. — Thomas Jefferson

When we get piled upon one another in large cities, as in Europe, we shall become as corrupt as Europe.
— Thomas Jefferson

The democracy will cease to exist when you take away from those who are willing to work and give to those who would not. — Thomas Jefferson

It is incumbent on every generation to pay its own debts as it goes. A principle which if acted on would save one-half the wars of the world. — Thomas Jefferson

I predict future happiness for Americans if they can prevent the government from wasting the labours of the people under the pretence of taking care of them. — Thomas Jefferson

My reading of history convinces me that most bad government results from too much government.
— Thomas Jefferson

The tree of liberty must be refreshed from time to time with the blood of patriots and tyrants . . . — Thomas Jefferson

Banking institutions are more dangerous to our Liberties than standing armies. If the American people ever allow private banks to control the issue of their currency, first by inflation, then by deflation, the banks and corporations that will grow up around the banks will deprive the people of all property until their children wake up homeless on the continent their fathers conquered.

— Thomas Jefferson, 1802

It is impossible to maintain a free society when more and more people look to the state to provide what Americans used to provide for themselves. — Warren Pollock

Capitalism gave the world what it needed, a higher standard of living for a steadily increasing number of people.

— Ludwig von Mises

To the masses, the catchwords of Socialism sound enticing...so they will continue to work for Socialism, helping thereby to bring about the inevitable decline of the civilisation which the nations of the West have taken thousands of years to build up. — Ludwig von Mises

Under capitalism the common man enjoys amenities which in ages gone by were unknown and therefore inaccessible even to the richest people. — Ludwig von Mises

To assign to everybody his proper place in society is the task of the consumers. Their buying and abstention from buying is instrumental in determining each individual's social position. — Ludwig von Mises

No currency can hold up in the face of an economy that survives on borrowed money and debt. — Richard Russell

No one would remember the Good Samaritan if he'd only had good intentions. He better had money as well.

— Margaret Thatcher

Government is so big today that more than half the population gets a major part of its income from the state.

— John Stossel

Paper money has had the effect in your state that it will ever have, to ruin commerce, oppress the honest, and open the door to every species of fraud and injustice.

— George Washington

The state is no organism capable of bringing either moral or material improvements to the populace, but merely a vehicle of power for the men and party in power.

— Niccolo Machiavelli

The fall of a great nation is (almost) always a suicide.

— Arnold Toynbee

Civil liberties, once so easily and thoughtlessly surrendered, will be harder by orders of magnitude for our children and grandchildren to reclaim. — James R. Muhm

Government today, far from protecting property, is its main threat. — Roger Pilon

In a social democracy with a fiat currency, all roads lead to inflation. — Bill Fleckenstein

What a government system can accomplish is to destroy the art and science of medicine in these United States of America.

— Jane M. Orient, M.D.

What is called the "private sector" of the economy is, in fact, the voluntary sector; and what is called the "public sector" is in fact, the coercive sector. — Henry Hazlitt

Short-sighted and impatient efforts to wipe out poverty by severing the connection between effort and reward can only lead to the growth of a totalitarian state, and destroy the economic progress that this country has so dearly bought.

— Henry Hazlitt

[I]t is a paradoxical truth that tax rates are too high today and tax revenues are too low — and the soundest way to raise revenues in the long run is to cut rates now.

— John F. Kennedy

John Kennedy once said to an assembled group of scholars in the White House, "I think this is the most extraordinary collection of talent, of human knowledge, that has ever been gathered at the White House — with the possible exception of when Thomas Jefferson dined alone.

Consumption never creates wealth. — Kurt Richebacher

The government has nothing to give to anybody that it doesn't first take from someone else. — Henry Hazlitt

If you think health care is expensive now, wait until you see what it costs when it's free. — P.J. O'Rourke

The costs of government are bound to be much higher than those of the free market. . . . The state cannot calculate well and therefore cannot gauge its costs accurately.

— Murray N. Rothbard

The way to crush the bourgeois is to grind them between the millstones of taxation and inflation. — Lenin

I am for doing good to the poor, but I differ in opinion of the means. I think the best way of doing good to the poor, is not making them easy in poverty, but leading or driving them out of it. — Benjamin Franklin

The greatest danger to the liberal vision are facts about the consequences of liberalism itself and the laws, policies, and ways of life that the left has spawned. That the black family, which survived centuries of slavery and generations of discrimination, has disintegrated in the wake of the liberal welfare state is only one example. — Thomas Sowell

History shows that people who save and invest prosper, and the others deteriorate and collapse.

— Jim Rogers

Abused and neglected children have paid the price for liberalism's tendency to sentimentalise the poor.

— Mona Charen

There is one, and only one, social responsibility of business — to use its resources and engage in activities designed to increase its profits so long as it stays within the rules of the game, which is to say, engages in open and free competition without deception or fraud. — Milton Friedman

The past seventy-five years have seen the growth of government from a relatively small entity charged with defending the borders, adjudicating disputes, and delivering the mail, to a bloated nightmare creature whose tentacles reach into every corner of our existence.

— Doug Hornig

We were poor when I was young, but the difference then was that the government didn't come around telling you, you were poor. — Ronald Reagan

A government which robs Peter to pay Paul can always depend on the support of Paul. — George Bernard Shaw

I believe the money I make belongs to me and my family, not some governmental stooge with a bad comb-over who wants to give it away to crack addicts for squirting out babies.

— Andy Rooney

If the bureaucracy is not checked, it will tend to build . . . in the name of peace . . . a defence against every conceivable contingency; so much "security" that "the secured" are without resources . . . helpless and hopeless.

— Leonard E. Read

The world's most powerful investment bank [Goldman Sachs] is a great vampire squid wrapped around the face of humanity, relentlessly jamming its blood funnel into anything that smells like money.

— Matt Taibbi, *Rolling Stone* magazine, June 2009

Fiat money, in extremis, is accepted by nobody. Gold is always accepted. — Alan Greenspan, May 1999

While the crash only took place six months ago, I am convinced we have now passed through the worst — and with continued unity of effort, we shall rapidly recover. There has been no significant bank or industrial failure. That danger, too, is safely behind us.

— Herbert Hoover,
President of the United States . . . May 1, 1930

It is well that the people of the nation do not understand our banking system, for if they did, I believe there would be a revolution before tomorrow morning. — Henry Ford

On every continent, and in every epoch, the peoples who have excelled in creating wealth have been the victims of some of society's greatest brutalities. — George Gilder

Money, when considered as the fruit of many years' industry, as the reward of labour, sweat and toil, as the widow's dowry and children's portion, and as the means of procuring the necessaries and alleviating the afflictions of life, and making old age a scene of rest, has something in it sacred that is not to be sported with, or trusted to the airy bubble of paper currency. — Thomas Paine

Part - II
Essays in Contemporary Economics

In Gold We Trust

THE purchasing power of the dollar has been declining ever since it went off the gold standard in 1971. When we look at every paper dollar note, one dollar note to 100 dollar note, there is an inscription, In God We Trust. The founding Fathers of America had a strong belief in both God and gold as the real money, and the dollar was always anchored to either gold or silver or both. In fact, it was illegal to counterfeit the currency, anchored to gold, in any manner, punishable by the penalty of death. The belief of only gold as money was so strong, they could have printed GOLD in place of GOD.

During the Great Depression, every major currency abandoned the gold standard. This pattern repeated throughout Europe and North America. In the US, the Federal Reserve was forced to raise interest rates in order to protect the gold standard for the US dollar, worsening already severe domestic economic pressures. After bank runs became more pronounced in early 1933, people began to hoard gold coins as distrust for banks led to distrust for paper money, worsening deflation and depleting gold reserves.

In early 1933, President Roosevelt implemented a series of Acts of Congress and Executive Orders which suspended the gold standard except for foreign exchange, revoked gold as universal legal tender for debts, and banned private ownership of significant amounts of gold coin. These actions were upheld by the US Supreme Court in the "Gold Clause Cases" in 1935.

The next politically popular option, to stabilise falling prices, was to devalue the dollar on foreign exchange markets. Under the Gold Reserve Act the value of the dollar was fixed at $35 per ounce of gold, making the dollar more attractive for foreign buyers. This change led to more conversion of gold into dollars, allowing the US to effectively corner the world gold market. Under the post-Second World War Bretton Woods system, all other currencies were valued in terms of US dollars and were thus linked to the gold standard. The need for the US government to maintain both a $35 per troy ounce market price of gold and also the conversion to foreign currencies caused economic and trade pressures. By the early 1960s, compensation for these pressures started to become too complicated to manage.

In March 1968, the effort to control the private market price of gold was abandoned. A two-tier system began. In this system all central-bank transactions in gold were insulated from the free market price. Central banks would trade gold among themselves at $35 per troy ounce but would not trade with the private market. The private market could trade at the market price and there would be no official intervention. The price jumped to $43 per troy ounce. This gold price increase turned steep through 1972 and hit a high that year of over $70. By that time floating exchange rates had also begun to emerge, which indicated the *de facto* dissolution of the Bretton Woods system. The two-tier system was abandoned in November 1973. By then the price of gold had reached $100 per troy ounce. In the early 1970s, inflation caused by rising prices for imported commodities, especially oil, and spending on the Vietnam War, which was not counteracted by cuts in other government expenditures, combined with a trade deficit to create a situation in which the dollar was worth less than the gold used to back it.

In 1971, President Richard Nixon unilaterally ordered the cancellation of the direct convertibility of the US dollar to gold. The sudden jump in the price of gold after the demise of the Bretton Woods accords was a result of the significant prior debasement of the US dollar due to excessive inflation of the monetary supply via Federal Reserve. In the absence of an international mechanism tying the dollar to gold via fixed exchange rates, the dollar became a pure fiat currency and as such fell to its free market exchange price *versus* gold. Consequently, the price of gold rose from $35 per troy ounce in 1969 to over $500 in 1980.

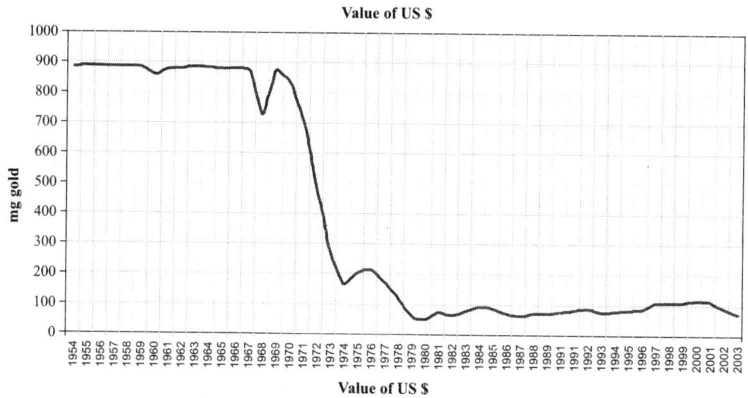

This graph shows the final closing value of the US dollar for each calendar year. Value is measured in milligrams of gold. The dollar was worth about 80 milligram or $400 per Troy ounce in 2003. Today, gold at $1660 per ounce, the dollar buys less than 20 milligram.

Shortly after the gold price started its ascent in the early 1970s, the price of other commodities also began to rise. Fearing the emergence of a gold-based economy separate from central banking, and with the corresponding threat of the collapse of the US dollar, the US government approved several changes to the trading on the Commodity Exchange. These changes including the exorbitant interest rate charged on borrowed dollars, resulted in a steep decline in the traded value of precious metals from the early 1980s onward.

However, as the economy started to stabilise, the free market economy started to flourish, with falling interest rates. The return on equity started to rise and the stock market exploded. The Dow Jones index went from around 800 in 1982 to over 11,000 in the year 2000. However, in hindsight, it was also due to a technology bubble and the cheap fiat dollar. New financial products, in form of derivatives, also came into the market and the total notional value of these products started to rise exponentially. Rulers of the Western governments started to believe in ingenuity of their rocket scientists who had developed these new derivative products. That also brought calamities in developing countries like Malaysia and Indonesia depressing their currencies. The yen carry trade in 1998 illustrates how overinvestment and near unanimity of market opinion can lead to a vicious squeeze. Whoever could borrow yen at near zero interest rate borrowed yen and then converted into currencies that yielded much higher return, assuming that the exchange rate remained stable. However, a very high demand of yen made yen more valuable with respect to high yielding currency. The squeeze got initiated on yen borrowers as yen kept rising, and the currencies that were sold started falling.

Something similar to the yen was initiated in the year 1999, when every banker of the country's central bank wanted to lease or sell unyielding gold assets to generate cash flow. Discarding deeply rooted tradition based upon the experience of thousands of years is dangerous. John Maynard Keynes had the right idea about gold as an inelastic currency. However any idea at the extreme will not work for long — it is the sweet spot or the middle portion of the pendulum swing that keeps us safer. A perception had developed among central bankers with total unanimity that the stored gold held as a national treasure was a dead asset.

Following the 7 May 1999 announcement that the United Kingdom (UK) would sell more than half of its gold reserves, gold and gold shares plummeted. The UK sale came out of the blue and could not have been more perfectly designed to damage investor confidence in gold and gold shares. Still, gold shares remained above their August, 1998 lows, thereby refusing to confirm the new 20-year lows set by the metal itself. A major bear trap was set in, one that was several years in the making. Mining companies in particular expanded in an orgy of hedging since the UK announcement. The rush to the exits when the bearish case became front-page news was consistent with odd lot behaviour and a good omen that a major low was in place.

Gold's breakdown was based on two incorrect beliefs: first, that all central banks will sooner or later sell all of their gold; second, that the best of all possible worlds of that period regarding inflation and financial markets will last forever. It was nothing less than capitulation to financial market euphoria. The value of all financial stocks had risen from an average of 10 per cent during previous decades to around 30 per cent in the year 2007. The gold market had already absorbed vast quantities of unreported selling that dwarf announced outright bank sales. A significant percentage of the borrowed or leased gold had already been melted down and sold into the physical markets. Physical gold borrowed from the central banks had been sold over and over again in multiple transactions. Through the magic of derivatives, paper claims had multiplied against a shrinking base of physical gold. Over 10,000 tonnes of central bank gold had disappeared forever. It represented about 35 per cent of the total reserves of the 80 or so central banks known to lend gold. The transaction occurs among three parties, central banks, bullion banks, and mining companies.

In a forward sale, a mining company directs the bullion bank to sell a certain quantity of gold for future delivery. The bullion bank borrows gold from a central bank for a very low gold lease rate, and sells the gold into the physical market. At that moment the bullion bank is short. The expected repayment of the gold is from future production of the mining company. Against one spot sale, two claims arise. The central bank has a claim on the bullion bank. The bullion bank has a claim against the mining company's future production. Two short positions arise from one physical transaction. In the world of options and hedging, the leverage to physical gold far exceeds the two to one of a simple forward sale.

What can go wrong? First, the mining company may be unable to produce the gold. Second, the lease rate charged to the bullion bank could rise sharply, as it has in the past, and wipe out their profitable spread. Third, gold could rise suddenly and sharply, triggering margin calls from the central bank to the bullion dealer. Fourth, local currency fluctuations could undermine economics of the hedge. Fifth, sovereign risk considerations could substantially alter credit quality.

About 12 years later, today we now know that the things did go wrong, and the price of gold has risen over fivefold. And the gold carry trade, I believe has not ended yet. What happened in 1999 was almost certain a bear trap, and the bear was indeed trapped. With all the uncertainties in currency markets, the bullish trend should last until the dollar is stabilised. However America has no choice but to devalue the dollar to come out of the deep hole of debt. President Obama declared in his January 2010 State of the Union Address that he would like to increase the export by 100 per cent. Only way that can be done is by cheapening the dollar, so that the Boeing planes and other products become cheaper to export. Using the year 1980 as a reference for the gold peak price of about $800 per ounce, and the money supply of today and of 1980, the next peak price of gold should occur around $8000. If we were to take the real rate of inflation of about 7.5 per cent from 1979 onwards, the price of gold should be over $7500 per ounce. The hard asset expert Doug Casey calls the dollar as an *IOU nothing*, and euro as *who owes you nothing*. Gold, on the other hand, having no liability of any kind, owes us everything. The gold bull market, I believe, has years to go. Remember, central bankers were net sellers of gold for over 20 years, and have become buyers just last year.

What should be the price of gold by the end of December 2011? Looking at the data of last 8 years (2003-10), the summer low occurred during the period of 1 June through 12 August. The average maximum gain at the end of each year was 30 per cent. The summer low of $1485 occurred on 1 August. Then the price of gold should rise over $1930. However, JP Morgan Chase (JPM) made a recent statemennt that the gold price could go as high as $2500. JPM in my opinion did it to attract as many speculators as they could to trap them. As the price rose close to $1900, they pulled the rug and at the opportune time, dropped the price, since bullion banks are also the market makers. As of this writing (24 August), the gold price has dropped close to around $1700. It may take few weeks to stabilise before it starts moving up again. Market technicians believe that the spot gold should bottom around $1675. Following the same process for silver, the year end price of silver should be around 50 to 55 dollars.

My good friend Anand Rao Lingayat sent me following two *shlokas* from *Mahabharata*, page 535, Khanda 6 (महाभारत: अनुशासनपर्वः दानपर्व).

पवित्र च पवित्राणाय मंगलानां मंगलम्।
यत् सुवर्णं स भगवानअग्निरीशः।।

Gold is the most auspicious among the auspicious
and the luckiest among the lucky;
gold is Agni — the God of fire himself and the Lord himself.

पवित्राणां पवित्रं हि कनकं द्विजसत्तमाः।
अग्नीषोमात्मकं चैव जातुरपमुदहृतम्।।

Gold is the holiest of the holy, it is considered
the avatar of the God of fire and the Sun

So if gold represents the God of Fire in our Indian tradition, then it is not too farfetched to interchange GOD and GOLD on a dollar currency notes.

The Economist magazine predicted in 1988 that a new currency named *Phoenix,* a bird rising from the ashes, will replace the dollar by 2018. What else can rise out of ashes but gold? Gold is money, nothing else. Gresham's law states that the bad money (overvalued) drives out the good money. So the good money, gold, is stored, while the fiat money is in circulation. Eventually, the bad money dies, and out of the ashes rises the *Phoenix,* probably a gold or silver backed dollar or a currency accepted by multiple nations — something which could happen in a decade or two.

August 2011

Anthropocene
The Age of Man

THE earth is huge with its 7 billion inhabitants. Humans have become a great force of the nature, in reshaping the planet on a geological scale at a far-faster than geological speed. A single engineering project, the Syncrude mine in the Athabasca tar sands in Canada, involves moving 30 billion tones of earth — twice the amount of sediment that flows down all the rivers in the world in a year. Geologists look at the distribution of fossils, at the traces of glaciers and changes in sea-level, and at other forces that have shaped the planet. Now a number of these scientists, based upon the editorial of *The Economist* magazine dated 28 May, are hypothesising that future geologists observing this moment in the Earth's progress will conclude that something very odd was going on. Scientists are increasingly using a new name for this new period. Rather than placing us still in the Holocene, a peculiarly stable era that began around 10,000 years ago, the geologists say we are already living in the Anthropocene: the age of man. The Anthropocene is different. It is one of those moments where a scientific realisation, like Copernicus discovery that the earth goes round the sun, could fundamentally change people's view of things. It means more than rewriting some textbooks. It means thinking afresh about the relationship between people and their world. Too many scientists embrace that the nature can be studied in isolation from the human world, with people as mere observers. There is no more objective truth of Einstein

— we, humans matter, more than ever in the past. Subjective truth of Tagore is becoming more relevant. Textbooks will have to be re-written if archaeologists discover that Indus civilisation was older than the civilisation of Mesopotamia.

The sheer amount of biomass now walking around the planet in the form of humans and livestock, handily outweighs that of all other large animals. The world's ecosystems are dominated by increasingly homogeneous crops, livestock and creatures, that get on well in environments dominated by humans. Creatures less useful or adaptable don't survive: the extinction rate is running far higher than it was during normal geological periods. A planet, that could soon be supporting as many as 10 billion human beings, has to work differently from the one that once held just 1 billion people, mostly peasants, only 200 years ago. This outward expansion, or the cultural evolution of the last 200 years, external to the human body, is due to the creative order-generating activity of the human mind, as I have described in my book, *Transcendence: Saving Us From Ourselves*. This cultural evolution (or a revolution), is much faster than natural evolution. Tools such as mathematics, language, and modern hardware, make these processes predictable. Biological, meaning somatic evolution, is natural, unpredictable, and not accessible to the human mind.

The characteristics of a Heraclitean (ancient Greek philosopher) view of Nature, closer to views expressed in Indic tradition, are: Nature is running down in energy, but running up organisationally, with ever more information and wisdom. There is an end state of every order that results in chaos and anarchy, producing total disorder. However, there are steps we humans could take to slow down the process going towards the end state. For example, maintaining autonomy at every layer of a dynamic system, while adjusting to the changing environment, prolongs the life of the system.

The challenge of the Anthropocene is to use human

ingenuity to set things up so that the planet can accomplish its planetary functions in the twenty-first century. Quite small things, such as smarter farming and better sewage treatment, could help a lot. It is possible to add to the planet's resilience, often through simple actions, if they are well thought through. One message of the Anthropocene age is that piecemeal actions can add up to planetary change, prolonging human existence on the planet. However, there are plenty of negatives, natural and manmade, that could be detrimental to human survival. William Huston, a specialist in natural and human behavioural cycles (author of the book, *Future Storm . . .*, 2003) describes six different dynamics which could cause un-surmountable calamities. At least four of them seem to be materialising.

These six dynamics are: Terrorism associated with religion that could cause armed holy war. The worst case scenario would be jihadists acquiring nuclear arms. The second dynamic is due to cultural evolution associated with the information age. The worst case scenario is what we are witnessing today, namely, revolt and uprising in the Middle East and southern Europe. This is an index of planetary instability caused by rapid and widespread information dissemination and its political deployment, not a comment against democracy. The third dynamic is due to the changes in the weather patterns. This could lead to widespread famine, killing millions, as the effect of volcanic eruptions and absence of sun spots lowers the temperature by several degrees. The fourth dynamic is the cycle of disease; when there is no known antidote for pathogens like Ebola, millions could die. The fifth dynamic is due to the shortage of energy supply, causing a severe slow down of the economic machine. The sixth and the last dynamic is the bursting of the credit bubble. America has become the largest debtor country ever in the whole of human history. The worst case scenario is the demise of the dollar causing hyperinflationary depression.

Some combination of the above scenarios, like longer winters causing lower crop yield, with sky rocketing cost of energy, and over all unbearable inflation, could bring civil unrest in America, more violent than the one we see in Europe and north Africa. This period, in Huston's estimate, could last for decades. Barron's cover story (5 July 2011) about crude oil price rising above $150 per barrel, adds more fuel to the fire. America has even more problems to resolve. Currently (22 July) both parties are log jammed in matters of raising debt ceiling.

The debt could keep rising if no action is taken by the government. The most menacing culprit is the rising cost of medical benefits due to the rising population of baby boomer retirees, and rising average age due to the advancement in medicine. There has been a perception that we can maintain our standard of living just by innovation. If we use our minds, we do not have to produce any hardware in a factory. Some economists would say about Asia and America that, "we think and they sweat". I would like to counter this by saying, "we must sweat, think, and introspect" for our well-being. There would be more people earning better wages in manufacturing than those employed in service industries. Wealth is created by producing more, not by consuming more. We should never stop being creative and come up with ideas that give us a better life. But, we must go even further and enter the realm of philosophy and introspection to come at the threshold of spiritual self and by learning to practise austerity.

We have heard about peak oil, peak water, and peak food implying that these commodities will become scarcer in time because the production cannot catch up with consumption. Yes, it is likely that it could happen since more people in developing countries would like to have the same lifestyle as those in the West. Then, there are three peaks that go hand in hand, peak consumption, peak greed, and peak stupidity. Over consumption is one of the causes of obesity. Why don't we have peak caution, not peak greed? I suppose greed caused the bursting of the credit bubble predicted by William Huston, resulting in the 2008 financial meltdown. We have no choice but to go in to the process of deleveraging. The pendulum has changed the direction from extreme greed and consumption towards caution and hopefully saving for a rainy day. Adapting to changing environment, together with austerity and introspection for the growth within will go a long way for the good of humanity and the mother earth.

One day, America will lead the world to climb the mountain of austerity. Austerity here does not mean asceticism, but simpler living, avoidance of waste, and being environmentally friendly. Climbing a mountain is not an easy endeavour. America may have to descend a little, go around the obstacles as long as the direction is towards the mountaintop. The day America is at the mountaintop of austerity, will be a day to celebrate. We will be in harmony with nature around us, harmony of body, mind, and spirit.

July 2011

Anekantavada
The Truth in Matters of Economy, Markets, and Money

TRUTH is something that all cultures claim to revere, but perhaps we fear it as much as we desire it. I find it intriguing that one of the oldest fragments of the Christian Gospels that sits in a museum in Dublin, is a piece of parchment from the Gospel of John dating to the second century CE. The fragment quotes Pontius Pilate as he confronts Jesus: And Pilate asked: "What is Truth?"

Humanity, it seems, is always looking for the truth. But perhaps we play lip service to the term and don't want to know it. Is it because "truth" is tough to bear? The Roman Catholic Church had difficulties in accepting Galileo's truth that the earth is round. We have an expression in India: *Satyameva Jayate — "victory is always to the truth."* Mahatma Gandhi revered the word so much that he titled his autobiography "My Experiments with Truth". In the introduction he states: "I worship God as Truth only. I have not yet found Him, but I seek him. I am prepared to sacrifice things dearest to me in pursuit of this quest, even if the sacrifice demands my very life."

Western philosophers view truth in different ways employing different theories, like *correspondence theory*, *coherence theory*, *consensus theory*, *pragmatic theory*, *pluralistic theory*, *redundancy theory* and so on. They often separate formal, that is, mathematical truth from historical truth. The Eastern and Western approaches to discover the truth are quite different. Western view in essence is Einstein's objective truth based upon intellectual non-hindering observations. The current state of materialism is probably at the highest level due to the scientific discoveries humanity has made. The truth of science, materialists believe, comes closest to the absolute truth unless it is proven untrue. The implication here is that even materialists would have to agree that there is no such thing as *absolute* and *forever* unchanging truth in nature. Einstein's discovery of *Relativity* rendered *Newtonian Mechanics* limited. The Eastern view is Tagore's truth based upon subjective experience; it is unique but never absolute. Recall the experience of the blind men of Hindustan and an elephant or the Jain concept of **Anekantavada** (or Anek Vad, that is many sidedness, or many paths to the mountain top). Philosopher Alfred Whitehead seems to agree with the Indian view. He states, "There is no whole truth; all truths are half truths. Treating them as the whole truth is to play with the devil". Immanuel Kant, perhaps due to the influence of eastern traditions, views truth as determined by employing all human faculties including intellect and intuition.

So what are the **Anekantavada** currently in matters of main street political economy, markets and money? The debt of over 14 trillion dollars is a big albatross around the neck of the American economy. There are three ways to get out of the debt in general. One way is to grow out of the debt as we do in leveraged real estate; as the rents go up, the burden of the mortgage diminishes. Another way is an outright default. The third way, also known as financial repression, is by devaluing the dollar employing inflation. For example, 5 per cent rate of inflation for ten years knocks down the value of debt from 100 to about 60. The Fed would like to tackle the debt burden employing both higher GDP growth and a controlled but higher rate of inflation keeping the interest rate close to zero. So far the Fed does not seem to have achieved either of them. The GDP growth is very weak, and the desired rate of inflation, in wages is close to zero. In fact, there is inflation in undesirable places obstructing the growth of GDP; the price of energy and commodities are rising inflicting pain to every household.

This is how I interpret what analyst Clive Maund had to say about Fed. The Fed is aware of its loose money policy pushing the dollar ever closer to the abyss and towards a painfully high rate of inflation. He believes that they engineered a financial system which essentially turned the rest of the inhabitants of this planet into servants of the United States, with their reserve currency status for the US dollar, and have cajoled the rest of the world into handing over its savings to be used to support a sumptuous standard of living in the US and a big military to police the globe in furtherance of US interests. He also implies that the Fed and Too Big to Fail banks engineered the 2008/09 market meltdown to prop up the dollar and the Treasury market.

The Fed is expected to wheel out quantitative easing #3 (QE3) in a timely manner. They may not do it immediately. The first thing that will happen is the threat of higher interest rates that will cause the commodity markets and stock markets to tank. Commodities and stocks have not been doing well lately because there is no real economic recovery, much less because of genuine demand for end use. They were going up earlier because of the huge leverage employed in these markets by speculators, who have been borrowing money at zero or near zero rates and pyramiding speculative positions. As soon as these markets perceive a threat to the supply of cheap money they will tank and the drop will be magnified by margin calls. The Fed can achieve this result by stating that it is not going to do QE3, and then do it anyway a little later to save its cronies in the big Wall Street banks from the threatening consequences of a derivatives implosion. When they do QE3 after all, the commodities and stocks road show can get rolling again. Just imagine how much money will be made by the elites who are in on this game plan. What we have described is a hypothesis, but the first whiff of it would certainly explain the bearish action in commodities during the first few weeks of May. A reporter asked Bernie Madoff sarcastically when he was taken to the jail," how do you fill about becoming the operator of the largest Ponzi scheme ever in the history?" Madoff replied," No, I am not the one, the largest operator is Uncle Sam".

This is what Mark Mobius, a famed fund manager of emerging markets, had said about derivatives: "*There is definitely going to be another financial crisis around the corner because we haven't solved any of the things that caused the previous crisis*". The main culprit will again be derivatives, whose effective regulation has been repeatedly stymied by the major financial houses. They make a heck of a lot more money designing and peddling these financial products and employing a high frequency trading algorithm when the clients can't quite figure out their true market value or the risks they entail.

Before the US housing bubble burst, securitised debt and derivatives accounted for roughly 80 per cent of global liquidity and amounted to about five times global GDP. Derivatives totalled about $350-trillion before the crisis. Since then, derivatives have grown to about 10 times the world GDP. As derivatives expert Satyajit Das has warned, if a bunch of big banks, interlinked through derivatives, run into serious trouble again, we'll be staring at another disaster. "*Derivatives will play their traditional part, which is communicating the risk at the speed of light. And in the period of history that we have just gone through, nobody has corrected anything. So we don't have any more circuit-breakers than we did then.*" Making matters worse, the surviving too-big-to-fail banks are bigger than before the crisis. Mark Twain once observed: *"It is not worthwhile to try to keep history from repeating itself, for man's character will always make the preventing of the repetitions impossible."*

Often I wonder why America would buy resources from other countries and restrict American companies within their own boundaries. Buy natural resources, like oil, with worthless fiat dollars as long as it can. Drain out resources of other countries, before they extract what is within their land. If and when other countries realise what America has in its planning, the end result will be nationalisation of their own natural resources. The ultimate outcome would be much higher prices of precious natural resources.

Who is the greatest enemy, perceived by America in particular, and by the West in general? This question was asked to Julian Assange of the Wikileaks. His answer was music to my ears . . . he said it is Ignorance, the view held in our Eastern scriptures. As I have expressed often, the good and evil (or the God and Devil) are a pair of opposites, where the evil is ignorance or the darkness and the good is the truth or the light. The darkness is also lies and misinformation propagated by ambitious politicians and their surrogates in the news media. One of the most important discoveries made by humanity is the Internet, and cellphones. However Nature always creates the opposite, not only of good things of life but also of bad things. The Internet is also the tool of the power-hungry empire builders. They use it for spying and spreading lies for their advantage. Facebook, Google, and Yahoo, all provide automated interfaces for America's Intelligence community free of charge.

Professor Debashish Banerji's Response on Anekantavada

On the subject of Anekantavada, this is the Jain philosophy based on ancient Sankhya, which believed there is one *prakriti* but many *purushas*. The Gita modifies this view by saying that the idea of many *purushas* is an illusion of ego. Gita postulates ego, *ahamkara*, as an attrribute of *prakriti*. Since *prakriti*'s attribute of *ahamkara* makes us experience oursleves as separate, we believe there is radical plurality, *anekantavada*. But if one realises this and overcomes ego, then one finds that there is One Purusha or *Purushottama* who has become all the beings of this world. The Gita asserts it is possible to have the experience of the One Purusha, which each of us is and all of us are, by eradication of ego and grace of God. But when we speak of it, we will return to relativity and speak of it differently. This is also the meaning of the Vedas' statement "The Truth is One, the sages speak of it differently" (*ekam sat vipraha bahudha badanti*). The story of the four blind brahmins and the elephant from the Upanishads deals, on the other hand, not with wise men (*vipra*) but with blind men, that is ignorant men, men who believe in their separate existence due to the existence of *ahamkara*. If they overcame this blindness, they would no longer be blind, they would see the elephant as one reality. They may still describe it differently, but each would understand that what the other said was another description of the same. This is because *purusha* is the knower, *prakriti* is the expresser.

11 June 2011

Versatile Silver, a Poor Man's Gold

PRECIOUS metals, particularly silver (poor man's gold) took a dive, down about 27 per cent from the peak, in the first ten trading days of May. However, the long-term bullish trend has not changed. Investment trends, based upon mass psychology, can be compared with tides, waves, and ripples occurring in oceans. Tides are caused by the planetary gravitational forces and of longer duration. The price decline in the month of May was more like a wind-generated ocean wave that got dispersed only in ten trading days. The tidal price movement for gold and silver has years, maybe a decade, to go. Just to get the long five-year perspective of the big picture, please note that, the price of silver, gold and S&P 500 are up 175 per cent, 130 per cent, and only 2 per cent respectively. I have explained in several articles going back to 2004, presented in this space and posted at www.nalandainternational.org, why precious metals should maintain a tidal bullish trend.

A fascinating article was published in the 1980 September issue of the Playboy magazine (PBM) and well worth the read for anyone interested in the silver market, its versatility, and restlessness due to human greed. A short synopsis of the story is that the Hunt brothers bought so much silver in the mid to late '70s that they nearly cornered the market. They bought 55 million ounces in late 1973 and early 1974 at around $3-$4 an ounce and sent 40 million ounces of it by chartered plane to Switzerland because they feared the US government would confiscate silver in the same way it had stolen gold from US citizens in the 1930s.The rationale for their buying made perfect sense. Nixon had taken the dollar off the gold standard, so dollar was now a purely fiat currency. The Hunts feared that their wealth was going to be stolen by the printing presses and they wanted to protect their immense inheritance from their father, who had made billions in oil.

They continued buying for years and even went into partnership with some Arab Sheiks. They set up a Bermuda-based trading company called *International Metals Investment Company Ltd.* The firm listed four principals: Nelson Bunker Hunt, William Herbert Hunt, Sheik Mohammed Aboud Al-Amoudi and Sheik Ali Bin Mussalem. This firm was incorporated in the summer of 1979 just prior to the immense spike in silver. They bought 90 million ounces of silver through the partnership and also wanted to take delivery of the silver. The silver price spiked sharply from $8 to $16 during August and September 1979. The commodity exchanges were worried that they would not be able to make delivery of silver when they came due.

This is where it gets really interesting. And we can see some parallels to the current price action in silver . . .

As stated in the PBM article, "The boards of both the Chicago and the New York exchanges were composed not only of 'outside' directors but also of representatives of the major, usually Eastern-based brokerage houses. Later testimony would reveal that nine of the 23 Comex board members held short contracts (meaning they sold silver at a higher price to buy back later at lower price) on 38,000,000 ounces of silver. With their 1.88 billion dollar collective interest in having the price go down, it is easy to see why Bunker did not view them as objective regulators."

As the price of silver continued to climb, the regulators began changing the rules. First the Chicago Board of Trade (CBOT) raised the margin requirement and declared that silver traders would be limited to 3 million ounces of futures contracts. Traders with more than that would have to divest themselves of their excess futures holdings by mid-February 1980.The price of silver really started to shoot to the sky because there was a perceived silver shortage. By the end of 1979 the price stood at $34.45.

On January 7, 1980 the Comex changed the rules again. The exchange announced new position limits for futures contracts of 10 million ounces. The effective date for the limits was February 18, 1980. After this announcement, the price climbed higher and the Hunts kept buying. On January 17 silver hit $50 an ounce. On January 21, the Comex announced its *coup de grace,* saying that trading would be limited to liquidation orders only. The exchange changed the rules so that no one was allowed to open any new positions from that point on. You could only liquidate open positions. Fed chairman Paul Volcker had kept on raising the interest rate (over 12 per cent) to subdue a very high rate of inflation. He was also liquidating government stock pile of silver. The next day silver fell off a cliff and plunged from $44 to $34.

The price of silver kept falling and the Hunts couldn't cover their margins on the futures they had bought. The Fed stepped in for fear that a huge financial panic was about to ensue and lent $1.1 billion to the Hunts to cover their margins but demanded a huge collateral for the loans. Nelson Bunker Hunt could not pay back the loans, and eventually went bankrupt in 1988.

Today, 30 years later, the silver price has once again scaled the heights to $50 an ounce. The exchanges changed the rules favouring bullion banks, to increase the margin requirements. The outcome was the plunge in the price of silver by 27 per cent in a week ending May 6th 2011. There are rumours that JP Morgan (JPM), one of the bullion banks, holds an immense short position in silver that was feeling the pinch.

What better way for them to relieve the pressure than to turn the screws on the long positions by raising the margin requirements substantially so as to then pick up the pieces at their leisure? After reading the history of the Hunt brothers and seeing that the futures exchanges change the rules of the game after the fact, you have to view the current price action in silver with a little more scepticism.

In 1980, the fall was due to the exchange's desire to hurt a big player who was long. Today's move, I believe, is more about protecting the position of *Too Big to Fail* insider (JPM) who is short and hurting. The recent price drop is a reaction only and cannot be compared to that of 1980 since the circumstances are entirely different. We have an ingrained systemic problem with Greece like financial balance sheets. We have the spectre of OTC derivatives that only grows and grows, preventing any Volcker type move. The cost of money (real interest rate) in 1980 was in double digits, compared to today's negative real interest rate. Besides Quantitative Easing has a cumulative bullish effect on precious metals.

Therefore, the chances are high that the price of silver should once again scale the heights if the players who are short use this sell-off to cover their short positions. There is still a lot of pent-up demand for precious metals and central banks continue to print. In fact, the buyers in Asia and particularly in India have resumed buying more after the price drop of almost 30 per cent.

During depression years, as described by Roy Jastram in his book, *Silver, The Restless Metal,* the miners were ready to sell silver for pennies. America was then holding over four billion ounces of silver. In 1939, professor Murad of Rutgers

University wrote silver's epitaph: *"No one has any interest in silver, except those unfortunate enough to be mining this unwanted commodity"*. America had over two billion ounces of silver in 1969; the treasury, during the ten year period, sold 93 % of the stockpile to greedy contractors and bankers to maintain the price of silver suppressed. About 139 million ounces were left at the end of the year 1979. All the remaining stockpile was gone by the end of the year 2000. Please note that the price of silver has gone up from about $4.5 in the year 2001 to over $30 per ounce today.

Billionaire Hugo Salinas Price, a very influential Mexican, predicts that Mexico may anchor the Mexican peso to silver. If this does happen, it will be extremely bullish for silver. I would not be surprised to see silver trade in some trading range for a few months during this seasonally weak period for metals and after taking such a hammering. There will be a time in the next few months when silver should become a bargain again.

May 2011

Silver, Opium and Paper Dollars

THE Opium Wars of 19th century, as described by Professor Fekete of Romania University, do not belong to the glorious episodes of Western history. Rather, they were instances of shameful behaviour the West still has yet to acknowledge.

In an effort to curtail silver continuously leaving mercantile governments (290 thousand tonnes from the mid-17th century) as payment for the Chinese goods (tea, silk, porcelain), Britain started the exportation of opium and tobacco with Spain and France following shortly after. America approved of these actions, claiming protection of free trade. Considering the danger of opium's addictiveness and potential to spread quickly in popularity, the Chinese ruling Dynasty prohibited selling or smoking the contraband in 1729 barring only minimal medicinal usage. But the damage had already been done, with China the dependent consumer of opium.

And, indeed, the flow of silver was first stopped, and then reversed. China was forced to pay silver for her addiction to opium smoking that was artificially induced by the pusher — the British.

The British endorsed smuggling despite China's wishes, and from 1773 to 1838, exports grew from 15 tonnes to 1,400 tonnes, almost a 100-fold increase in 100 years, forcing China to initiate the death penalty for trafficking. China attempted to regain control by confronting related British facilities and boarding their ships in international waters to stop the opium from reaching Chinese ports. Britain unjustly retaliated by claiming the Chinese had destroyed British property, catalysing the first opium war by intruding upon China with their superior British-Indian army. After Britain used warships to attack towns and take over tax barges, severely depleting China's income, China had little choice but to sue for peace in1842. Before the treaties were implemented with the US and the French, the Nanking Treaty set an example by demanding China pay Britain, open its port cities for which British subjects would have extraterritorial privileges and cede Hong Kong to Britain.

After the first War, things were only moderately quiet until 1856 when the Chinese searched a suspicious-looking British ship, and Britain used this event as an excuse to take over and later occupy the port city of Canton. China, the victim country, had no choice but to sue for peace once again with the British and the French. The Tianjin peace treaty called for China to create 10 new port cities, pay three million ounces of silver to Britain, two million to France, and allow free foreign passage throughout China. This deliberate humiliation of China by Western powers contributed greatly to the loosening and ultimate snapping of the internal coherence of the Qing Dynasty, leading to the Taiping Rebellion (1850-1864), the Boxer Uprising (1899-1901) and, ultimately, to the downfall of the Qing Dynasty in 1912. The American president, John Quincy Adams, chimed in during the debate by suggesting that opium was a "mere incident". According to him "the cause of the war was the arrogant and insupportable pretensions of China that she would hold commercial intercourse with the rest of mankind not upon terms of equal reciprocity, but upon the insulting and degrading forms of the relations between lord and vassal."

I recall the 1963 movie, *"55 Days in Peking"*, starring Charlton Heston, and David Niven. The movie is about the Boxer Uprising as viewed by the colonial powers. At the end of the movie, they show how the British-Indian army with tall Sikh soldiers saves the European diplomats and their families confined in their quarters. However, one dialogue between the Empress and the British diplomat is a reminder of the greed of colonial powers:

Empress: "13 of the 18 provinces of China are under control of colonial powers. Your warships and army occupy our harbours and forts, your merchants administer our banks. Your gods disturb the spirit of our ancestors. Is it surprising that our people are aroused? China is a helpless cow, the Powers are not content milking her but must also butcher her".

British diplomat: "If China is a cow, Your Majesty, she is indeed a marvellous animal. She gives meat as well as milk. . . ."

President Barack Obama's reaction to China's currency exchange-rate policy has been similarly disapproving for the same reasons as before, and China once more feels cheated for what it has received in exchange for Chinese goods. China has accumulated shrinking US treasury bonds denominated in dollars. The only difference today is the absence of opium in the dispute. The role of opium in the current dispute is played by paper, paper dollars, to be precise.

The accelerated demise of the dollar was initiated, decades ago, by the then President Nixon, when he disconnected the dollar from its anchor, gold. With no moral motivations to refrain from blatantly lying about where paper money would take the economy and the country, the paper dollar gained the desired reputation as the supposedly magic fix to the distresses of the times. This change served its real purpose in raising the paper dollar to the desired role of international currency. The fact that fiat paper money has a history of 100% mortality was neatly side-stepped. Any questioning of the wisdom of experimenting with it in spite of logic and historical evidence was dubbed as reactionary thinking.

The explanation for this self-destructive behaviour is the addictive and mind-corrosive nature of paper money, in direct analogy with that of opium. The "high", caused by administering the opium pipe to the patient, analogous to administering quantitative easing, or QE, had to be repeated when the effect faded by a fresh administration of more opium, that is QE2.

Today China, being sufficiently strong, will contest the force-feeding of paper money down its throat. This round differs in that China will not be the one to be humiliatingly defeated. China has been replacing dollars, as fast as it can, surreptitiously or otherwise, as it did before over 100 years ago, with gold, but more with silver. Please observe how the price of silver has skyrocketed in last couple of years, stronger than even gold.

There is another story about opium and the paper dollar that in some ways follows the law of karma. Ashish Nandi, an Indian philosopher and Gandhian, has proposed a theory of ethical cycles analogous to cycles of karma. It states that anything good done or bad inflicted by one nation or a group to another, in any field, returns to the giver or the inflictor in a cyclical movement of history. Nandi gives an example of the West exporting opium to China over a century ago, now the East exports the same to the West. I would like to extend the analogy further about opium and the paper dollars. In 1718, the College, established by clergymen in New Haven, Connecticut, was renamed *Yale College* (now University) to honour a gift from Elihu Yale, a governor of the *British East India Company*. It is also known that Mr. Yale, who donated dollars to build Yale University, made his money by selling goods including opium. Similarly, an Easterner, over a hundred years later, Mr. Ganpat Patel of Los Angeles has established a North Gujarat University, India, in the East, employing dollars earned in the West.

What do we learn from these historical events? I do not mean to regress, bringing to mind black thoughts of revenge. I simply would like to see more balance and harmony between the two opposites of a pair, the East and the West that would ultimately complement each other. More needs to be done to avoid polarisation and build more bridges between the pair. The modern world is dominated by a Western world-view, as a result of Western jingoism. But the legacy of the East has always been the power of knowledge. For a solution to inequalities, a clear perception of the problems is first necessary. It seems every pair, liberals and conservatives, labour and management, paper currencies and inflation hedges, and many more, all seem to be out of balance. Then there are problems of corruption at the highest levels in India and GAPONOMICS, implying widening gap between the rich and the poor in western countries, featured in the March 12th issue of the magazine, *The Economist*. What we need is life-education, not merely professional education without morality, which has led us to the exploitative world of today, but the education of the heart. I hope more emphasis is put on such education at every level. Just as opium and paper currencies have gone back and forth, now education that unifies humanity, but maintains individual autonomy, that stimulates the highest level of creativity, should become our universal currency, with hopefully more positive results.

March 2011

Broken Records of 2010 and Trends of 2011

2010 WILL be remembered for many events, but one that matters the most is the economic decline. Some of the records broken last year, collected from several sources, are stated below.

An all-time record of **2.87 million US households** received a foreclosure filing in 2010. The number of homes that were actually repossessed reached the **1 million mark** for the first time ever during 2010. The price of gold moved **above $1400 an ounce** for the first time ever in history during 2010. According to the American Bankruptcy Institute, approximately **1.53 million** consumer bankruptcy petitions were filed in 2010, which was up 9 per cent from 1.41 million in 2009. This was the highest number of personal bankruptcies we have seen since the US Congress substantially tightened US bankruptcy law many years ago. At one point during 2010, the average time needed to find a job in the United States had risen to an all-time **record of 35.2 weeks.** Back in 1970, 25 per cent of all jobs in the United States were manufacturing jobs. Today, **only 9 per cent** of the jobs in the United States are manufacturing jobs, which is believed to be a new record low. The number of Americans working part-time jobs "for economic reasons" was the highest it has been in at least five decades during 2010. The number of American workers that are so discouraged that they have given up searching for work reached an all-time high near the end of 2010. Government spending continues to set new all-time records. In fact, at the moment the US government is spending approximately **6.85 million dollars** every single minute.

The number of Americans on food stamps, and living in poverty **surpassed 44 million** by the end of 2010. This was a new all-time high in 51 years of record-keeping, and government officials fully expect the number of Americans enrolled in the programme to continue to increase throughout 2011. The number of Americans on Medicaid **surpassed 50 million** for the first time ever in 2010. According to the FDIC, **157 banks** failed during 2010. That was the highest number of bank failures that the United States has experienced in any single year during the past decade. The Federal Reserve brought in a record **$80.9 billion** in profits during 2010. They returned $78.4 billion of that to the US Treasury, but the real story is that thanks to the Federal Reserve's continual debasement of our currency, the US dollar, measured in purchasing power, **was worth less in 2010** than it ever had been before.

It is projected that the major financial firms on Wall Street will pay out an all-time record **of $144 billion** in compensation for 2010. Americans now owe **more than $881 billion** on student loans, which is a new all-time record. In July, sales of new homes in the United States declined **to the lowest level ever recorded**. According to Zillow, US housing prices have now declined **a whopping 26 per cent** since their peak in June 2006. Amazingly, this is even farther than the fall in house prices during the Great Depression. From 1928 to 1933, US housing prices only fell 25.9 per cent. State and local government debt reached at an all-time record of **22 per cent** of US GDP during 2010. The US national debt has surpassed the **14 trillion dollar mark** for the first time ever and it is being projected that it will soar well past 15 trillion during 2011.

After the tumultuous years of the Great Recession, a

battered people may wish that 2011 will bring a return to kinder, gentler times. But that is not what is being predicted. Instead, the fruits of government and institutional action – and inaction — will ripen in unpleasant outcomes. Trends that have been brewing for some time, should reach maturity in 2011, impacting just about everyone in the world.

So what are the trends projected for 2011? **Gerald Celente of Trend Research forecasts the following trends.**

Wake-Up Call: In 2011, the people of all nations will fully recognise how grave economic conditions have become, and how ineffectual and self-serving the so-called solutions have been. Having become convinced of the inability of leaders and know-it-all "arbiters of everything" to fulfil their promises, the people will do more than just question authority, they will defy authority. I believe pure democracy hardly exists in a few countries. In America, we have plutocracy, ruled by bankers and power elites. Egyptians are enjoying the downfall of Mubarak in the name of democracy, but the military is unlikely to let go of the power they now hold.

Crack-Up 2011: The reliable indicators (employment numbers, the real estate market, currency pressures, sovereign debt problems) all bordered between crisis and disaster. In 2011, with the arsenal of schemes to prop them up depleted, Celente predicts "Crack-Up 2011": teetering economies will collapse, currency wars will ensue, trade barriers will be erected, economic unions will splinter, and the onset of the "Greatest Depression" will be recognised by everyone.

Crime Waves: No job + no money + compounding debt = high stress, strained relations, short fuses. In 2011, with the fuse lit, it will be prime time for Crime Time. When people lose everything and they have nothing left to lose, they lose it. Hardship-driven crimes will be committed across the socioeconomic spectrum by legions of the on-the-edge desperate who will do whatever they must to keep a roof over their heads and put food on the table.

Crackdown on Liberty: As crime rates rise, so will the voices demanding a crackdown. A national crusade to "Get Tough on Crime" will be waged against the citizenry. And just as in the "War on Terror," where "suspected terrorists" are killed before proven guilty or jailed without trial, in the "War on Crime" everyone is a suspect until proven innocent.

Alternative Energy: In labouratories and workshops, scientific visionaries and entrepreneurs are forging a new physics incorporating principles once thought impossible, working to create devices that liberate more energy than they consume. I believe natural gas will come into play in a much bigger way.

Journalism 2.0: Though the trend has been in the making since the dawn of the Internet Revolution, 2011 will mark the year that new methods of news and information distribution will render the 20th century model, that is Journalism 1.0, obsolete. With its unparalleled reach across borders and language barriers, "Journalism 2.0", incarnated in 21st century and associated with cyber-journalism, using transnational social media platforms, has the potential to influence and educate citizens in a way that governments and corporate media moguls would never permit.

Cyberwars: In 2010, every major government acknowledged that Cyberwar was a clear and present danger and, in fact, had already begun. The demonstrable effects of Cyberwar and its companion, Cybercrime, are already significant — and will come of age in 2011. Equally disruptive will be the harsh measures taken by global governments to control free access to the web, identify its users, and literally shut down computers that it considers a threat to national security.

Youth of the World Unite University degrees in hand, yet out of work, in debt and with no prospects on the horizon, feeling betrayed and angry, forced to live back at home, young adults and 20-somethings are mad as hell, and they're not going to take it anymore. Filled with vigour, rife with passion, but not mature enough to control their impulses, the confrontations they engage in will often escalate. Government efforts to exert control and return the youth to quiet complacency will be ham-fisted and ineffectual. The Revolution *will* be televised, blogged, YouTubed, Twittered.

End of The World! The closer we get to 2012, the louder the calls will be that the "End is Near!" There have always been sects, at any time in history, that saw signs and portents proving the end of the world was imminent. But 2012 seems to hold a special meaning across a wide segment of "End-time" believers. Among the Armageddonites, the actual end of the world and annihilation of the Earth in 2012 is a matter of certainty. Even the rational and informed that carefully follow the news of never-ending global crises, may sometimes feel the world is in a perilous state. Both streams of thought are leading many to re-evaluate their chances for personal survival, be it in heaven or on earth.

In matters of investment, market is telling us that silver may become one of the best insurances to protect our wealth. The housing market has not settled yet, since fore-closers have been increasing early this year. I do not anticipate a market crash since financial institutions, with the support of the government and The Fed employing derivatives, are managing and controlling the stock market at desired level with some growth even at the expense of higher inflation rate. This is the most desired solution in their mind to satisfy both public and private pension funds. There is plenty of cash on the sidelines that could still be deployed. Portfolio insurance is actively being purchased, which makes stocks less vulnerable to panic-selling when negative headlines hit the newswires, and short sellers are still actively engaged in the market — pressuring stocks coincidentally, but providing short-covering potential in the future.

In addition to the above trends, web surfing has helped me to discover the technological trends that are a result of the explosion of information humanity is experiencing. Please note that the wisdom is derived by braiding knowledge, distilled out from information, with experience.

India has more honour roll kids than all the kids in America, thanks to IIT and many more educational institutions. 25 per cent of all the workers in America have been working for less than a year with their current employer. Last year, 12 per cent of all married couples met online, thanks to web surfing. MYSPACE, with 200 million users would become the 5th largest country, if it was a country. The number of monthly searches on Google has exploded to 31 billion, ten times the number in the year 2006. It took 38 years for the radio to find an audience of 50 million. It took only four years for the Internet to find the same. It is estimated that forty million trillion (40 with 18 zeros added) unique units of information will be generated this year alone, which is more information than was generated in the last 5,000 years.

February 2011

A Picture is Worth a Thousand Words

IN mathematics, we speak of opposites in terms of digital (arithmetic) and analog (geometric). We often employ both tools to communicate a concept. An artist would recite a modified Shakespearian statement that the *world is an analog stage*, emphasising that the human mind is used more for understanding, grasping, absorbing and acquiring information on an analog plane rather than a digital one. Remember the saying, "A picture is worth a thousand words"? A picture is a display of information in analog form, while the words or captions beneath it can be counted and are therefore digital. Pictures and words, the analog and the digital, are pairs of opposites, but they work together in balance and harmony to inform and educate. Notice that two opposites don't have to be equal. To be sure, good and evil are not equal, although I, an optimist, believe that perceived good is in greater demand than a perceived evil in every society.

The trend has been established in the 21st century to convey and communicate in quick, short bursts. As a result, modern communication focuses on pictures, audio, and video rather than written words. This trend is the cause of more newspapers going out of business. It is also an indication of the contracting attention span of an average reader, or an increasing poverty in the time domain, meaning less time and more things to do. 50 per cent of the population in America obtained the news from newspapers in the early 1990s. Today it has shrunk to below 30 per cent and is declining.

Corporations have discovered that the written word is failing them. British Petroleum's spewing out into an open ocean on You Tube sent a message to the world far more compelling than any written statement ever could. Images get stuck in memory. Recall Walter Cronkite's sombre expressions and tearful eyes as he conveyed the death of President Keennedy. And the image of a self-immolating Buddhist monk on TV that changed the course of the Vietnam War. E-mail will still exist to communicate at work and among friends and family, but not for long as a means for mass communication, thanks to the firewalls created to reject advertisement. There will be a time when the pendulum will swing in the opposite direction, when words will take their rightful place.

In this article, dear reader, I will review, space permitting, a few currently published charts, audios, videos, and cartoons and interpret and convey the message focused mostly on the economy and Fed Chairman Bernanke.

A cartoon depicts the Fed Chairman Bernanke as Dr. Strangelove, who describes to President Obama with certainty how the economy will recover after the 2009 meltdown. One would have to see the movie, *Dr. Strangelove,* starring Peter Sellers, to understand and appreciate the message. It is a joke on the economic establishment. Like any monopoly, the economic establishment will try hard to suppress any view from the outside. A hundred years ago Max Plank, commenting on the resistance among physicists to the revolutions of relativity and quantum mechanics, joked that "science progresses one funeral at a time." The achievement of economists has been dismal, if not disastrous, in the last couple of decades. I suspect the cause of underachievement or failure may be due to associating more with hard science and very little with human psychology. As stated in *The Economist* magazine, the field of economics must reform itself quickly or the funeral will be for the discipline as a whole.

Ben Bernanke in a recent interview on CBS *Sixty Minutes* programme said the following:

> Well, this fear of inflation, I think is way overstated. We've looked at it very, very carefully. We've analysed it every which way. One myth that's out there is that what we're doing is printing money. We're not printing money. The amount of currency in circulation is not changing. The money supply is not changing in any significant way. What we're doing is lowering interest rates by buying Treasury securities. And by lowering interest rates, we hope to stimulate the economy to grow faster. So, the trick is to find the appropriate moment when to begin to unwind this policy. And that's what we're going to do.

This statement will probably go down in history as a greater folly than Gordon Brown's justification for the disposal of half of Britain's gold reserves right at the bottom of the gold market. Bernanke is printing massive quantities of money, which he here denies, and expects us to believe that the inflationary consequences are "way overstated". Yes, government data shows that the latest CPI is below 2 per cent. However, the cost of essential commodities that includes food and energy has gone through the roof. The bar chart reproduced by Casey Research shows that the yearly price of wheat, oats, pork and cotton has gone up over 60 per cent, while the price of canola, sugar, copper, heating oil, gasoline, coffee and beef has gone up over 20 per cent. It is pure delusion to say there is no inflation risk. In reality, there is inflation and deflation co-existing side by side. But Bernanke, like Greenspan, has to walk a tightrope, and he must realise that, though there are inflation risks, there have to be greater priorities, or undeclared reasons for printing money in such unprecedented quantities.

The two likely reasons are the perilous state of government finances and the potential for a second banking crisis. These problems are on a collision course, with the US economy and its tax base stalling on the edge of an economic abyss, and the banks trapped between rising domestic insolvencies and the consequences of the approaching Euro-land banking implosion. The Fed is nervously watching broad money, which has been contracting for about two years in spite of zero interest rates. Bernanke equates money with credit: he is expanding the money supply to counteract the contraction of credit. Apparently, Bernanke is more frightened by systemic problems associated with the contracting economy and deflation today, than by inflation tomorrow.

Americans are in no mood to support a second rescue package for the banks, so such a failure cannot be allowed to happen. The Fed, for itself and the financial system, is trying hard to have as low a public profile as possible: like a swan, serene on the surface while paddling furiously under water. However, the Fed has come under public scrutiny, having been recently forced to disclose to whom it lent money to resolve the first banking crisis. The yet-to-be-confirmed appointment of Ron Paul to the chairmanship of the Financial Services Sub-committee, which oversees the Fed, can be expected to force more disclosures and make Bernanke's life more difficult, more high-profile.

Jim Rickards, a prominent economist, recently gave a presentation in a conference about the economy and national security arranged by the Department of Applied Physics at John Hopkins University. He has come up with a conclusion and a solution to the current currency war, debt and deflation problems of Western countries employing dynamic systems analysis. There was unanimity in the conference that the current debt and deflation problem is lot more dangerous than any future terrorist attack.

The equation he uses for analysis is: MV=PY, where M is the money supply, V is the velocity of money, P is the price index, and Y is the growth rate. He reasons that when the Fed pumps in the money (M) in the form of quantitative easing or buying the treasury bonds, the Fed anticipates the growth rate (Y) to go up. However, the real growth rate is not going up because the velocity (V), that is money circulation, is not going up. Money stays in banks since they do not lend and businesses do not borrow because of uncertainties. He believes that sooner or later, increasing M could cause P to explode, meaning the rate of inflation could go out of control.

He believes that sooner than later, the world monetary system needs to get anchored back to gold as it had been for 5,000 years before 1971, when President Nixon disconnected the dollar from gold. If that does not happen, the world economy will experience periodic instability, getting more catastrophic in time, as it has happened in varying degrees in the last several decades. America, with the support of G-8 countries, could declare the dollar reconnected to gold at some future date when the conversion to gold can be determined. America, even today, has the advantage of holding the most gold, about 8,400 metric tonnes. America also has additional gold of Germany and a few other countries. Added all together including IMF gold, America could control as much as 18,000 metric tonnes of gold. Rickards estimates that the conversion could be in the range of $5,000 to $7,000 per troy ounce based upon the current money supply and other variables. He believes that even today currencies are connected to gold indirectly and the current price of $14,00 per ounce is very deflationary.

It is interesting to note that what is happening today with the weakening dollar and the street riots in Europe was depicted in a 1981 movie, *Rollover,* starring Jane Fonda and Kris Kristofferson.

(Articles of Mr. Doshi, a writer, trader and philanthropist, are available at www.nalandainternational.org)

Below are (two supporting articles from the Barron's Magazine.)

By Manuel Hinds

It is ironic that the international monetary system of floating currencies is based on a theory called the "Optimal Currency Area" that celebrates the freedom of central banks to print money at will. The idea is that total freedom to create money would promote global progress and employment, smooth out business cycles, and prevent bubbles and their associated crises.

The irony is that the system is obviously suboptimal. It goes against the grain of globalisation, the process that is defining our economic times. To accommodate the central bankers' wishes to control their own currencies, the floating system requires splitting the world's monetary markets into as many currency areas as there are countries.

This introduces a grave fragmentation in the international monetary markets precisely when all other markets, including the financial ones, are coming together into a single global market. It creates obstacles for the operation of the emerging global chains of production as well as for the international allocation of resources. Fragmentation also opens the door for currency and financial crises, turning capital flows, a naturally stabilising force, into a destabilising one through currency speculation.

Unbridled monetary printing led us to the collapse of Bretton Woods in the late 1960s and then into the stagflation of the 1970s and early 1980s. Then, after a brief recess that ended in the mid-1990s the result of Paul Volcker's refusal to print money during his tenure as Federal Reserve chairman — we returned to trigger-happy monetary creation.

As a result, in the past 15 years we have gone from bubble to bubble, and from bust to bust, printing money first to keep the economy going; then to overcome the bursting of the dot-com bubble, then to sustain a triple bubble of housing, securitised instruments and commodities; then to overcome the effects of the bursting of these bubbles, which is leading to a second commodity bubble and a boom in emerging markets that seem to be waiting to go bust. It is as if we believe that by printing money we can remove hard budget constraints.

Worse, as happened in the mid-1930s, when currencies also floated, countries are engaging in currency wars that nobody can possibly win. The objective of all warriors is to depreciate their currency more than the rest of the world. In the process, while all currencies are debased, the floating system is failing to perform its most elementary promise: absorbing international imbalances. As with the United States and China, the absorption of these balances has ceased to be based on automatic, economic processes and has become the subject of political confrontations.

This failure should lead us back to the drawing board to re-design the international monetary system, reversing the trend that prevailed during the 20th century. We started that century with a fundamental international currency, gold, which kept its value through time and was widely accepted around the world. We ended the century with more than 150 currencies that change their value constantly and at different rates from each other, in such a way that most currencies are not accepted in most countries.

In pursuance of the illusion that money can remove hard budget constraints, we moved from order to disorder. After demonetising gold in the 1970s, now we are demonetising money by debasing and politicising it.

Mentioning the gold standard that prevailed all over the world during the Industrial Revolution brings about derisory comments, some of them suggesting that the value of gold was based on fetishism. This is a mistake. The gold standard was a highly rational system. It kept prices constant through centuries and provided an automatic mechanism to remove international imbalances, such as those that are creating today's currency wars, without the help of any international bureaucracy.

The gold standard achieved this not because of any mystical property of gold itself but because it was an impersonal system. Central banks or governments could not tamper with monetary creation. This is what we need today.

Mr. Hinds is the former finance minister of El Salvador and the co-author of *Money, Markets and Sovereignty*, which won the Manhattan Institute's 2010 Hayek Prize. This op-ed is adapted from Mr. Hinds's remarks upon receiving the Hayek Prize.

The Beginning of The End of Dollar Hegemony

By Randall W. Forsyth

With nascent use of other currencies for finance, will redbacks replace greenbacks?

When the monetary history of the year coming to an end is written decades from now, the headlines of European debt crisis and Federal Reserve's adoption of QE2 may turn out to be mere footnotes to the bigger story: 2010 could be a watershed marking the beginning of the end of the dollar-based, Western-centric monetary system.

To be sure, suggestions that the system dubbed Bretton Woods II should be supplanted by a new regime began in 2009. China proposed the creation of a new, multinational currency for international transactions and as a reserve asset.

This year, the idea of reform was advanced by World Bank President Robert Zoellick, who proposed in a widely read and commented-upon *Financial Times* op-ed piece "a cooperative monetary system that reflects emerging economic conditions." That would include the dollar, the euro, the yen, the pound and the renminbi — plus gold "as an international reference point of market expectations about inflation, deflation and future currency values."

Zoellick's November commentary followed the outbreak of the so-called "currency wars," as Brazil's finance minster dubbed the tensions in the foreign-exchange markets resulting from Fed's liquidity expansion through the purchase of $600 billion of Treasury securities, dubbed QE2, for the second phase of quantitative easing. The downward pressure on the dollar from the surfeit of greenbacks was viewed by finance officials abroad from Asia to Europe as well as Latin America as tantamount to a competitive devaluation to boost the US economy while beggaring its neighbours.

The ire aroused internationally by QE2 has been compounded by events that demonstrate there really is no ready substitute for the dollar as an international reserve currency. The hope had been for the euro to provide a viable alternative to the dollar, and for a time, the single currency seemed to grow into that role. Prior to the financial crisis of 2008-2009, for a time more global bonds were issued in euros than dollars.

But the European sovereign debt crisis has resulted in what German Chancellor Angela Merkel called "serial bailouts" of first Greece last spring and now Ireland. The current crisis lays bare the contradictions that have beset the euro from the start: monetary union without fiscal union, not to mention nationalistic animosities going back decades, even centuries. How long the serial bailouts can paper over these things remains to be seen.

Dissatisfied with the options of the dollar or the euro, the ascendant economic powers are essentially cutting out these middlemen. Only recently, Micex, Russia's largest securities exchange, began trading in the rouble vs. the Chinese renminbi. It was largely symbolic, given the volume traded was equal to about $700,000. More importantly, Russia and China have agreed to settle their bilateral trade of about $50 billion in their respective currencies.

That means Chinese importers don't need to obtain dollars to buy oil from Russia. Nor does Russia need greenbacks to buy Chinese goods. The vast majority of international trade has been, and continues to be, conducted in dollars.

Financial markets also are dominated by dollar instruments, even if they trade in London or Singapore or any number of financial centres around the world. But less so than before.

It used to be that if an emerging market such as Brazil wanted to borrow, it would have to issue dollar-denominated bonds because of lack of international confidence in its currency, which had been devalued and replaced numerous times over the year. Now, Brazilian government bonds denominated in the real are so sought after by international investors for their double-digit yields in an appreciating currency that the government has put a tax on foreigners wanting to buy the securities.

But the biggest development has been in the burgeoning in so-called dim-sum bonds — securities denominated in renminbi by non-Chinese borrowers. Issuers include blue-chip US corporations such as Caterpillar (ticker: CAT) and McDonald's (MCD.)

That's a huge, but largely underappreciated development. Because the rest of the world uses the dollar for transactions and a store of value, the US has been able to take advantage of that. Indeed, the greenback is America's most successful export.

So, Americans get the goods, allowing us to consume more than we produce, simply because the rest of the world wants our paper. That fuels the US credit expansion that covers the gap between Americans' savings and US investment, including for residential real estate. Without money from abroad, there would not have been the housing bubble. American ingenuity produced triple-A mortgage-backed out of subprime loans, which dollar holders around the globe eagerly scooped up.

These foreign dollar holders are funnelling their funds into Treasury securities, effectively funding the US budget deficit. But they're not doing it as willingly as before. The *Financial Times* reports that some Chinese have taken to calling the renminbi the "redback," in contrast to the American greenback, which gives some idea about the competition between the currencies is playing out.

None of this suggests that the dollar is about to be toppled from its perch as the premier global currency in 2011. Strains in the original Bretton Woods system were evident long before President Nixon abrogated the promise to redeem dollars for gold at $35 an ounce for foreign monetary authorities on August, 15, 1971. Even then, the floating exchange-rate system didn't come into being fully until 1973.

China is keeping a tight rein on the renminbi. Its exchange rate is held down by China's policy of buying dollars to keep the RMB in check. Those dollars eventually are recycled into US assets.

How long this process goes on depends on the availability of alternatives to the dollar. Direct settlement of trade in the currencies of trading partners cuts into demand for dollars, as does the availability of investments such as renminbi-denominated dim-sum bonds.

When the tide changes, the shift is almost imperceptible. The tides of history are by nature very long term. The last great sea change came when the dollar replaced the pound-sterling as the world's main reserve currency. The dollar's role was cemented under the Bretton Woods Agreement following World War II, when other currencies' exchange rates were fixed in terms of the dollar and the dollar was convertible into gold at $35 an ounce.

Since 1973, the dollar has been unanchored and has been anything but a stable store of value. Based on the US Dollar Index — which measures its value in terms of a basket consisting of the euro, Japanese yen, British pound, Swiss franc, Swedish krona and the Canadian dollar — has risen from its 1973 base of 100 to as high as 140 in the 1980s and 120 in 2002 to a low around 74 in early 2008 as the financial crisis deepened. It currently hovers around 80.

The components of the Dollar Index seem almost quaint as they ignore the BRIC countries — Brazil, Russia, India and China. Back then, their presence was barely felt in the world economy. And the old world order persists elsewhere; Belgium and the Netherlands have greater voting rights in the IMF than China, now the world's second-largest economy after surpassing Japan this year.

Seen from a historical perspective, if the 20th century was the American century, it would be natural that the dollar wouldbe the dominant currency. The 21st century is being called the Asian century. Brazil is part of that, now that China is its main trading partner, overtaking the US. So, too, is Australia, which is booming as a commodities supplier to Asia.

The demand for dollars from the rest of the world has been of inestimable benefit to the US economy. It quite simply allows Americans to consume more than they produce and save less than they invest; in other words, to live beyond our means. The dollar's dominance will not be toppled in 2011 but will wane over the coming decade and beyond. And America will have to start picking up the tab for what had been a free lunch.

December 2010

Silver, India's Rupyak

THE term for silver, probably for it's beautiful lustre, also happens to lend its name to the currency of India, the rupee (Devanagari: Rupyak), since the dawn of human civilisation. In India, silver coins, associated with Goddess Laxmi, are given as gifts on auspicious occasions. Few are aware of the gradual disappearance of existing silver in the world, and even fewer people are aware of the resulting inevitable increase in the value of silver.

I wrote an article titled, "A Tale of Two Metals......", in August 2009 and posted it on www.nalandainternational.org. I had given three reasons that could propel the price of silver, about $13 per ounce then, to much higher levels. These three reasons, in short, were: the demand exceeding the supply, price of silver coming back to its historical level with respect to gold, and the loss of control over the price suppression by institutions in cahoots with the government.

Recently something has drastically changed in the silver market. Some banks that once participated in controlling the price of silver are now closing positions at a loss. The commercial shorts have begun to bleed money — and when blood spills, sharks will circle. Hedge funds and traders worldwide that never even thought of silver before will begin to squeeze the shorts. If the bullion banks, mostly American and English, don't quickly regain control of the silver market they may lose it forever. Yes, silver price was down by little over a dollar on October 19th, but that was after a steep rise from $17.6 to over $24 with hardly any significant correction. One way to measure the banks' hold on price control is to observe the difference between the silver spot price and the ETF or the paper silver price. The gap has been widening from 25 cents to over 55 cents over a period of less than a year implying that the deliverable silver is about 55 cents more expensive that the undeliverable paper silver. So the real retail cost of the deliverable silver, that includes retailer's commission, is about a dollar over the paper or the ETF silver (symbol: SLV) traded in the New York Stock Exchange.

Another measure of the bullion banks' hold on the price of gold and silver is to look at the history of the price, and calculate the product of the per cent drop in the price and the time interval it took to erase the drop. This product, calculated for gold, has been contracting steadily from about 1,700 units (per cent drop times weeks) in 2008-2009 to about 100 units in May 2010. The implication here is that the price drop, manufactured by bullion banks, are shallower and are not able to keep it for long. There seems to be a correction in precious metals that got started on October 19th. However, this correction should not be significant unless we fall into another deflationary cycle and the market crashes.

Anyone following the futures market for silver knows that the large commercial traders like JP Morgan (JPM), always win. That is until now. Let's look at the history of short selling as it is related to silver in the past, what has been occurring recently and what may unfold in the near future, as follows.

During the bull market in silver that began in 2001, a pattern of trading similar to the "Martingale Betting Strategy" emerged, in which 8 bullion banks sold short increasingly larger amounts of contracts into rallies, until their sales volumes overwhelmed the market into a freefall. After the freefall, they then repurchased those short positions at a profit and the rally process began again. This process of taking money from precious metals investors, has been well documented by analysts such as Ted Butler, David Morgan, and others. The strategy was so successful that some futures traders began to frontrun the banks on their own, using tactics such as the Commitment of Trader (COT) report and other sentiment indicators. As a result of their actions it has been argued that these large short positions have suppressed the price of silver significantly.

Until just about eight weeks ago (until August 20th) all was going according to plan. Silver rallied and the commercial banks shorted an ever larger amount of contracts as the open interest swelled to the point at which most silver analysts were expecting a correction. In the following two weeks silver rose by nearly $2 dollars and most were expecting to see an even larger commercial short position reflected in the COT report. Instead, the commercials actually covered 2,300 contracts, and bought an additional 990 long contracts during the week of September 28th to October 5th when the price of silver rose by about a dollar (tradeplacer.com). The covering was down at what appeared to be a short-term top to many.

While it can be speculated on how short covering could impact the market, a short squeeze could feed upon itself as it attracts capital. In five trading days of buying a net 3,286 contracts the price of silver rose by $1. However, the commercial banks are still a net 62,127 contracts short so at that linear rate it would take them 94 trading days to cover with a silver price of roughly $117. The resulting losses would be around $15 billion. Of course, markets are not linear and after the second or third week of covering, traders would begin to purposefully frontrun and squeeze the commercial shorts so it is unlikely that the positions could be covered that low or if at all. Potential buyers hoping for a correction to accumulate more silver may not get it here as the price may never get substantially lower. Please note that in the past two months silver has rallied 31 per cent — more than three times gold's 8.9 per cent rise.

In the modern age of instant communication, the whole world knows about the managed (manipulated) gold and silver market, and the out of control world reserve currency, the dollar. Countries like China are making legal and even encouraging the populace to hold gold and silver. Their leaders, claiming that we are now in a multi-polar world, want to replace the dollar with something else as the world reserve currency. Very recently China News Agency reported that China, one of the largest exporters of silver, will cut the export of silver by 40 per cent.

Investors in silver, also known as "poor man's gold," are persuaded by many of the same arguments that have driven the gold price higher: the prospect of a global "currency war" in which central banks race to devalue their currencies to support domestic growth and the belief that a second round of emergency monetary easing by the Federal Reserve could eventually lead to a sharp jump in inflation.

Precious metals and mining stocks represented anywhere from 20 to 30 per cent of the total global assets until 1981 (data available from 1921 to 1981). Today with rampant financial shenanigans and an elephant-size derivative market, this asset class is worth about one per cent of the total global assets. The price of gold keeps making all-time new highs, while the silver price today is still about 50 per cent of 1980 high of about $50 per ounce. It is apparent, at least in this writer's view, that silver has a great future even at this elevated price level.

In the meantime, the IMF was unable to stem the tide of competitive currency devaluations over the weekend of October 10th. As a result, governments and central banks around the world still have the green light to continue with their money-printing orgy. Some of the citizens of these various countries have recently been acting as their own central banks by purchasing gold and silver as insurance against the currency wars. As fears escalate, the question now becomes: when will the people of the world once again have stable systems of currency?

October 2010

Fault Lines; Saving Capitalism from Capitalists

I HAD an opportunity to listen to University of Chicago's Professor Raghuram Rajan when he was invited to speak at The Milken Institute in 2004 about his newly published first book, *Saving Capitalism from Capitalists*. He was then the chief economist of the International Monetary fund (IMF). The book comprehensively defends the free market system, steering a course between conservative isolationists and Left-leaning believers of anti-globalisation. He and his co-author Zingales, argue that unbiased, un-manipulated, free markets can provide an environment supporting competition, innovation and economic growth. The authors have harsh words for government interference through "subsidisation" or tariffs on foreign imports. Government support for the free market, they admit, is flimsy — not sufficient, particularly during economic down-turns. When markets are suppressed, as so happened after the Great Depression, competition is stifled and trade tariffs ultimately harm worldwide economic health — certainly in today's interconnected world. The authors, however, do advise economically advanced countries like the USA. to maintain a healthy balance between laissez-faire economic policy and government participation, providing measures of incentives for free markets and insurance for safety during times of crisis. It is important to note that successful capitalists often oppose the competition from new entrants into the market, as it happened in India immediately after independence, harming the Indian economy for decades. As I have argued in my book, *Saving Us from Ourselves,* the free market gives opportunities to all to prosper using their creativity and other God-given assets. When I raised the question about governments going back to the gold standard to control quantitative easing, Professor Rajan answered with strong conviction that governments will never let go their power of creating money.

Rajan's second book, *Fault Lines,* is possibly the most thought-provoking contribution in the aftermath of the 2008/09 crisis, which has not yet ended. Rajan argues that the initial causes of the breakdown were stagnant wages and rising inequality. With the purchasing power of the middle class household lagging behind the cost of living, there was a strong demand for money in order for an average American to survive. The financial industry responded by supplying home equity loans, subprime mortgages and automobile loans. The government supported these actions indirectly and often directly, without any concern about overextended leverage and credit growth.

The side effects of unrestrained credit growth turned out to be devastating — most economists, including the Federal chairman Greenspan, had failed to foresee such potential "Black Swans" arising. Fault lines along the tectonic plates of the global economy pushed big government, and "too big to fail" financial Institutions, into an unprecedented financial earthquake. Mr. Rajan, who had played Cassandra of the Greek Tragedy, had predicted in 2005 that the economy could falter, thanks to the economic imbalances — imbalances in trade deficits, imbalances creating extremes between the rich and the poor, imbalances due to government overspending, credit risk due to the housing bubble, sloppy US monetary management, and so on. Imbalance between two opposites of a pair, as I have argued, leads towards destruction.

Rajan, one of the speakers during the 2005 conference held at Jackson Hole, Wyoming, had the gall to stand up against the maestro Greenspan's parade with his gloomy predictions. A dubious audience, that included the maestro's cronies, did not think much of his analysis and predictions. When his words were finally proven true by the economic outcome three years later, he counselled that the financial world stop rewarding sub-par behaviour almost as greatly as superb performance and begin penalising failures, more strongly which were barely acknowledged at that point. Similarly in terms of necessary and appropriate repercussions, Rajan cautions his listeners about the continuation of a moral-hazard problem due to lack of consequences as a result of taking dangerous actions. Though he commends both the Bush and Obama administrations' handling of the bailouts in 2008 and 2009, he warns that if we don't make sure that the creditors, preferred shareholders, and financial-insurance customers of, say, AIG suffer substantial losses, the lack of consequences will result in a deception in matters of security risk.

Rajan believes the US, and especially Europe, have muted economic recoveries in store, based primarily on "Europe's sovereign-debt woes and the euro's decline". He warns that if the structural problems in the global economy continue to remain unacknowledged and unchanged, we will likely see more financial bubbles, and a global increase in severe credit blowups. This leads into his concern of the growing economic income gap, made clear by one of Rajan's cited studies that 58 cents of each dollar of wage growth went to the wealthiest 1% of households from 1976 through 2007 while the lower 50% have had a drop in incomes. Additionally, the US has a weak system of support for the unemployed with replacing 50% of the average loss in wages from 1989 through 1995, as opposed to Germany's 63% and France's 57%. Though France's benefits last up to three years, and Germany's up to 18 months,

US unemployment benefits are curtailed at 6 months and only *if the individual even manages to qualify for said unemployment.* Rajan reports that though lost jobs were recovered within eight months from 1960 to 1990, by 2001 the time it took to restore them had increased to a shocking 38 months. In a supposed effort to remedy this unemployment, the Fed utilised easy-money, low-interest-rate-policies, which resulted in greater proliferation of bubbles in commercial real estate and leveraged buyouts.

Rajan prefers the low interest rate to be a potentially great path of *only temporary* help for a wide spectrum of Americans without alienating conservatives through obvious income redistribution. With easy money, housing and the luxuries that follow become more affordable, which leads to an increase in related jobs concerning appliances, construction, mortgage finance, and the like. However, easy money policy for an extended period needs to be challenged. Considering the Fed pushed interest rates lower than optimal levels (from 6% to 1% between 2001 and 2003) due to fear of deflation and extensive job recovery, it's no surprise that Rajan's prophecy of the collapse of the housing bubble in 2006 and 2007 was unavoidable.

Rajan considers Greenspan's notorious 2002 speech to bankers in Jackson Hole the second great mistake of the central bank. Greenspan claimed in that speech that the Fed's purpose is to "mitigate the fallout and hopefully ease the transition to the next expansion," rather than taking on the responsibility of destroying asset bubbles, which earned the name, "the Greenspan put". The implication here is that if markets were to go chaotic, the Fed would step in to prop up prices and stabilise markets.

In Rajan's view, this emboldened the "cynical and amoral" producers of the mortgage securities to devise and peddle complex, hard-to-understand mortgage products that eventually proved toxic, and the short-sighted credit agencies to brand triple-A ratings on roughly 60 per cent of all asset-backed securities during the ensuing lending boom.

In Rajan's view, gross trade imbalances are another cause of a giant fault line. The US, known for being a great consumer, is relied upon by countries that focus on mostly export growth as opposed to internal demand, like Germany, Japan and China, to stimulate the market during times of economic duress. However, excess global supply ends up gravitating to countries having weak economic policies and little discipline. So countries like Greece and Spain keep spending to buy goods they may not need with money they do not have. Please note that these imbalances in the majority of Western countries could last for years to come.

After the Asian Flu period of 1997 to 1998, during which the East Asian nations' economies were deflated by an abrupt absence of foreign investment capital, these nations learnt well how large trade deficits can create tsunamis devastating their economies. As a result, many countries such as Malaysia, Taiwan, Korea, and Thailand have resolved to become net exporters of both goods and capital to the West, only adding to the global imbalances.

Rajan's experience in the global setting is not purely of book knowledge. As Rajan's father was an Indian diplomat, he was exposed to myriad countries and later obtained degrees in electrical engineering and management in India before obtaining his Ph.D. from MIT. Rajan is a walking, talking resource, utilised even by India's prime minister as an economic adviser.

August 2010

Economic Smor-Gas-Bord

THIS essay covers the current state of the economy, but not in a coherent, focused on only one view. I will look at the state of things and take snapshots at different angles. To start with, the economy seems to be in a state of deflation more so than inflation. One way to understand the mystery and give guidance to the future is through the crucial measure of the velocity of money. The velocity of money is the rate at which money changes hands, or how often a business may rotate its money. A low velocity of money, with decreasing sales and revenue, signals deflation. A high velocity with increasing revenue signals inflation. How do we measure it? The price of gold is one indicator. Recall the periods 1970 to 1980 and 2002 to 2007. When the price of gold stagnates, deflationary pressure dominates. Of course, it is more complicated than simply looking at the gold price alone. Another variable to consider is interest rates. If interest rates gradually rise, economic activity is also on the rise! The price of gold will keep rising if the rate of inflation is greater than the nominal interest rate. This happened in the 1970s. The price of gold will stagnate or fall if interest rates go substantially higher than the rate of inflation; this happened during the 1980's.

In the view of James Rickards, a prominent economist, we are experiencing a "natural" bout of deflation from the Great Recession and deleveraging. We are also experiencing "artificial" inflation from fiscal and monetary policy, zero interest rate policy (ZIRP) and quantitative easing (QE).The natural deflation and artificial inflation are offsetting each other so far, so that price indices are well behaved. But this is not price stability. Rather, this current situation is a mask for the temporary balance of the offsetting forces. Just because California is not shaking right now does not mean enormous stresses are not building below the surface and along the fault lines.

The problem for the Fed is that deflation is accelerating. This is what the bond market, with an interest rate close to zero, is telling us. The conventional response is more QE keeping ZIRP in place. But massive QE is not a free lunch. It can be as dynamically unstable as deflation. In particular, neither the Fed nor anyone else has a rigorous understanding of the volatility of velocity. Recall that if you double velocity, you double nominal GDP, assuming everything else remains constant. However, real GDP cannot grow annually at more than about 3-4% (i.e. population growth + productivity growth). This means that if velocity doubles and nominal GDP doubles, there will be, at best 4% real growth and the remaining 96% is inflation, which definitely qualifies as hyperinflation. The strongest correlation for inflation is between the money supply and credit expansion.

A massive increase in velocity, or the volatility of velocity, can cause a phase transition in the macro-economy from mild deflation to hyperinflation, analogous to when an overheated, boiling liquid turns into evaporated gas. That is exactly what happened in 1922 in Weimar Germany, when the value of currency evaporated to zero. So the policy question is: how much QE can the Fed implement before there is a loss of confidence in the value of paper money of the kind which will cause velocity to spike?

Economists anticipate that the Fed will fight deflation but will fear hyperinflation. As a practical matter, they will roll over investment in maturing bonds, extend duration, and engage in some new QE but not as much as they did very recently. In the short run, this will slow but not stop the deflation process. So there is potentially more room to rally in bonds. However, bond appreciation seems insignificant relative to the risk. But as nominal yields on bonds shrink, indicating continued deflation, the stock market should weaken further.

The most likely near term macro-economic scenario right now is a long period of little or no growth and mild deflation; i.e. exactly like Japan in the 1990s. But America is not as homogeneous as Japan and the US might have a very low tolerance for a continued deflation. Also, Japan's economy is export-oriented while 70 per cent of America's economy is based upon consumption. Political necessity might require that the Fed *"do something."* At that point, extreme QE could push the economy toward hyperinflation; in that event all paper debt assets begin to go to zero although select equities might get interesting again. Gold is still a winner, in deflation or in inflation. Investors need to be vigilant, agile and pull the trigger if and when necessary to protect the capital.

More evidence indicates that China is fighting the war against the West using the soft power. China apparently has given up using force since 1979 when they invaded Vietnam. It seems they no longer believe Mao's argument that "political power comes out of the barrel of a gun". They are using soft power quite skillfully. One example is giving low interest loans to African and Latin American countries. They have provided the largest contingent of soldiers for United Nations peacekeeping missions. They routinely manipulate their currency to keep prices of their exports artificially low. Beijing recently imposed a strict export quota of rare earth resources that are indispensable in high technology, e.g. for hybrid vehicles and computers. They have become the largest producers of gold and silver overtaking Africa and the Americas. China is increasing its gold reserve to strengthen its currency, though keeping its currency artificially lower to maintain and increase its exports. China has been very successful in outmanoeuvering the West whether at World Trade Organization (WTO), the United Nations, or other international organisations. They have done this by joining hands with BRIC (Brazil, Russia, India, including China) countries in matters of climate negotiations and the Doha trade talks.

History of World GDP (Casey Research Publication July 29, 2010)

	USA	China	India	Japan	W Euro.	Latin Am.	Other
1500 AD	0	25%	24%	3%	18%	3%	27%
1600 AD	0	29	23	2	20	1	25
1700 AD	2%	23%	24%	3%	22%	1%	25%
1800 AD	2	33	15	2.5	24	2.5	21
1850 AD	8	17	12	3	34	3	23
1900 AD	16	12	8	2.5	35	3.5	23
1950 AD	27%	5%	3%	3%	26.5%	8%	27.5%
2000 AD	22%	12%	5%	7%	21%	8%	2

As seen in the table above, the US ascendance occurred from 2% of world GDP in early 18th century (1700 AD) to 27% of the world GDP in 1950. China and India (Chindia) descended from 47% combined to only 8% of the world GDP during the same time span. However, the direction has changed during the last two decades. America's GDP with respect to the world GDP probably peaked some time in 1980/1990. USA's GDP dropped from 27% to 22%, while Chindia's GDP rose from 8% to 17%, more than doubling during the time span of 1950 to 2000. Western Europe's GDP also rose from 22% to 27%, and then back down to 21% in the same time span.

In matters of economy and markets, there are five major possible outcomes. First, we may continue on the path of slow deflation and declining money supply, Japanese style. The second and most desirable outcome would be moderate but controlled inflation with improving housing and the job market, and stable to slow rising interest rates. The most undesirable outcomes are the third, the fourth and the fifth which are Zimbabwe type hyperinflation, imploding depression, and the combination of both. Obviously, as I have explained in previous articles, gold in possession remains the strongest anchor during any of the five possibilities.

Seasonality and discouraging economic news about employment and housing do not bode well for financial markets. The market should perform better if and when the news about the economy and election results are favourable after the first week of November, 2012. That too could be short-lived.

August 2010

Revisiting Gold

Heads, I Win. Tails, Too, I Win

As all fiat currency systems over time have failed, our current one, too, is on a downward path. The dollar is trapped under the weight of almost $13 trillion in federal government debt and over $50 trillion in social security and unfunded future liabilities in Medicare. Our budget deficit remains over 10% of GDP as so many states approach bankruptcy. Currently, there is no other currency that can replace or compete with the dollar. As a result of Greece ready to default on its debt, Euro-zone members and the IMF have spent nearly $1 trillion to bail Greece out. Japan's government debt is already at over 200% of its GDP, and its rapidly ageing population is no help. After China's banks lent more than they could handle, the country is bearing the brunt of overcapacity, inflation and potential bad debt in the banking system.

After attempting to simultaneously keep the private sector from collapsing and bailing out the financial sector, the world's governments used widespread quantitative easing (money-printing) to fight deflation. The destruction of government balance sheets and the widespread implementation of zero interest rate policies may ultimately result in hyperinflation. We are experiencing simultaneously both deflation and inflation, deflation being a bigger problem for governments to overcome, due to credit contraction and the deleveraging process. Inflation is due to excessive money creation to fight deflation and the shortage of some goods and services like education and health care. Referring to Roy Jastram's book, *The Golden Constant,* holders of gold will preserve their wealth both in deflation and in inflation; hence the title of this article. He was able to prove, taking the data of the last 500 years, that the purchasing power of gold remains constant under all circumstances.

Jeffrey Christian of CPM Metals recently made known to the public that transactions on the London Bullion Market are minimally backed by available gold, though it is revered for reassurance of such gold's existence. Investors should be wary of paper gold products without the promised gold backing, gold ETFs, gold pooled accounts, and gold certificates which leave gold unallocated and therefore unaccounted for. Mine production has been steadily declining, while gold prices have been rising, suggesting insensitivity to high prices.

People seem to be ignoring the derivatives' role in the financial meltdown and the need to regulate OTC derivatives in spite of their being "financial WMDs". Their constant elevated notional value suggests either a major legitimate bet against the secular trend of gold prices or ongoing nefarious activity, such as serious price suppression. Price suppression's pre-existence is gaining increasing acknowledgement, partially due to the Gold Anti-Trust Action Committee (GATA), which has proven itself steadily accurate, though it has previously been ignored.

Aaron Regent, President of Barrick Gold, hinted in a conference that "peak gold" had already been met and can't be exceeded. The US is the world's largest gold holder, reported at 8,133 tonnes, and Germany holding about 3,400 tonnes. However, it is believed that Western central banks have employed swaps, leases and obscure accounting to covertly dispose of far more gold than they could in open market sale. Thus, leaving them unable to meet severe gold demands and so unable to keep the market in equilibrium.

Since the Feds have held off any audits since 1950, suspicions have arisen concerning this alleged US ownership of gold.

As the general populace becomes increasingly aware of gold as money, investment demand could potentially sky-rocket, resulting in new gold investment vehicles of unknown possibilities. India made known its purchase of 200 tonnes of IMF sale late last year around $1,050 per ounce, leading the charge to the gold world, with Russia, China and many other countries following with similar open intentions. Why is there so much interest in gold? Because, gold as money, is the most marketable means of exchange, chosen by unmanipulated free market.

The longest-established text-based religion in the West is about the God of Jacob — *His works and His worship*. For roughly five thousand years, a believer summed up his credo by saying, "I believe in God." But when this credo arrived, it had to share space with an alternative belief system that was almost everywhere in the world and was around for thousands of years before the Judeo-Christian era began. A believer in this system summed it up: "I believe in God." So we have two systems, and both are faith-based. It is difficult to prove to a sceptical rationalist why the tenet of God's belief is valid. However, gold has proven for millennia to be an everlasting, valuable, and stable asset to our wealth's protection.

As we contemplate this mental space sharing spiritual and temporal beliefs, we have mused that large-scale scepticism about both of them occurred only recently. Darwinism, palaeontology and astrophysics combined to drive the faith-related explanation of history out of the temples of scientific learning. Keynesian thought came along to drive gold from the temples of the central bank money-changers in favour of the printed paper promises of politicians. We do know that Nature's nature is to create pairs of opposite perceived by human mind. I strongly believe that the two opposite views in each pair can co-exist in balance and harmony, complementing each other, as it did when the paper dollar was anchored to gold for a century.

Future historians may well report that the moment when gold once again became a store of value was when the dollar began soaring in response to the stench of seared Greece — and gold climbed right along with it. The asset classes that have been inversely correlated since Keynes' time suddenly united. (Refer to articles posted at www.nalandainternational.org about gold and silver). As we have written in these pages, gold should retain its value under both inflationary and deflationary conditions. A great time to buy gold to make capital gains is when inflation is rising. It also means a great time to buy gold to conserve existing wealth when prospective risk-adjusted returns on bonds and stocks look unattractive, and also because the economic outlook is for slow growth with a risk of a renewed downturn that would hammer the value of stocks — particularly the financial and real estate sectors.

The bond yields are too low given the inherent risks in the currencies in which they are issued. The range of future fiscal deficit forecasts is from grim to ghastly. The supply of outstanding financial derivatives may be in the $70 trillion range, dwarfing the combined value of money supplies and debts. The total value of gold and gold stocks is so minuscule in comparison to the supply of these software-spawned instruments that it cannot be any real help in stabilising global finances, but it can be a haven for investors seeking to protect themselves against an implosion of majestic proportions.

In times of financial crisis, countries' bankers go back to gold because they lose faith in other currencies. France demanded gold for dollars in the early 1970s, and India, in 1991, had airlifted 47 tonnes of gold to London because it could not pay its debt in hard currencies of the time.

Is gold fairly priced? The long-term average house price has been about 350 ounces of gold. House prices were inflated at about 600 ounces during the 2006 housing market bubble. Currently one can buy an average priced house for about 150 ounces of gold ($180,000), implying that houses are cheaper than gold. However, with gold at $1,200 and Dow at 10,000, gold is cheaper than the stock market, since it takes a little over 8 ounces of gold to buy a Dow index. The long-term average is about 5 ounces. During the bear market bottoms of the 1930s and 1980s, one could have bought the Dow for less than 2 ounces of gold, implying that the Dow was dirt cheap. Some analysts believe that we could test the same level at the secular bear market bottom.

The long-term relationship of crude oil with gold has been about 20 barrels of oil for an ounce of gold. Today we get about 16 barrels, implying that gold is cheaper than crude. If we were to consider the relationship of gold with the quantity of money, depending on which money supply we use, the price of gold could be from $6,000 (M1) to $30,000 (M2) per ounce. Currently, gold has a much brighter future because of the excessive debt governments are carrying, maintaining close to zero interest rate on savings. A realistic target, based upon Elliot wave analysis is about $2,300. If and when interest rates skyrocket to control inflation, as it had happened in the 1980s, the price of gold could plummet.

Summing Up

> Browning said it (In *Rabbi Ben Ezra*), "Leave the fire ashes. What survives is gold".

The Economist magazine in 1988, predicted that a new currency named, *Phoenix*, a bird rising from the ashes, will replace dollar by 2018. What else can rise out of ashes but gold? Gold is money, nothing else.

July 2010

Derivatives
Lethal Financial Instruments of Mass Destruction

WARREN E. Buffett has warned over the past decade that derivatives are the fiscal equivalent of weapons of mass destruction (WMD). The consequences of an explosion of such a weapon could make the recent global economic crisis seem insignificant. But lobbyists, on behalf of big banks, plead for keeping the over-the-counter derivative market unchanged with no restrictions and no supervision.

Derivatives essentially are bets that come in different forms. Examples include a bet for or against the house in a casino, or against the weather in situations in which the weather is critical. Forwards, futures, options and swaps are different forms of derivatives. Credit derivatives are based on loans, bonds or other forms of credit. Over-the-counter (OTC) derivatives are contracts that are traded and privately negotiated directly between two parties, outside of a regular exchange. Just as the velocity is a time-dependent derivative of distance, so are the financial derivatives time-dependent. What happens between two parties, notably hedge funds, is like what happens between two individuals who bet on the final score of a football or baseball game. Congressional committees have been informed about "ticking time bombs" to no avail, demonstrating that both the US government and the US Congress are dysfunctional and out of sync.

On May 16, 2006, for example, Richard T. McCormack, Vice Chairman of Merrill Lynch and former Undersecretary of State for economic and agricultural affairs, spoke at a Senate banking hearing on derivatives and hedge funds in 2006, when the derivatives industry was in the $300 trillion range. He is quoted as saying "the increasing internationalization of finance and investment suggests the need for an ever-more-global approach to monitoring and controlling potentially dangerous problems." Derivatives played a key role in camouflaging the multibillion-dollar Enron scam in 2001. The Long-Term Capital Management (LTCM) hedge fund debacle of 1998 almost destroyed the global monetary system. Even though its trading losses were a mere $5 billion, it still threatened the soundness of the financial markets.

When the Russian rouble suddenly nosedived without warning, LTCM found itself exposed with more than $1 trillion in foreign-exchange derivatives it couldn't pay. The New York Federal Reserve Bank organised a consortium of companies to buy out LTCM and cover its debts. LTCM shareholders were wiped out, but none of the creditors took losses. LTCM was a hedge fund with just 200 employees, but without the New York Fed's intervention, it would have caused a crash felt around the world. Mr. McCormack pleaded with Congressional banking experts to correct any structural or technical problems that could increase the likelihood of systemic risk in the event of future shock to the financial system. There was no response from all the parties concerned, inside and outside the government. The 2007 US subprime mortgage global disaster was also derivatives-driven, and provoked the biggest financial and economic disaster since the Great Depression.

Mr. McCormack, then a senior fellow at the Center for Strategic Studies, explained to the Banking Committee how Italy had secured entry into the Euro by purchasing exotic derivatives that obscured the true financial condition of the country, until after they were admitted to the new European common currency. The same thing happened with Japan when some banks purchased derivative instruments, which disguised the actual catastrophic state of their balance sheets at the time. Today's massive new derivative bubble is driving the domestic and global economies, far outstripping the subprime-credit meltdown. Currently very few, "too-big-to-fail" banks, control the derivative markets and earn much more trading derivatives, employing their proprietary trading software, than from regular banking business. However, as more banks and hedge funds learn the same trick, it could culminate into generating more unpredictable and catastrophic "Black Swan" events. This is reminiscent of the morphic field described by Rupert Sheldrake in his book *The Presence of the Past*. He hypothesises that the rats in Europe learn the same trick, discovered by the rats in Asia, caused by this natural field analogous to an electromagnetic field. Please note that there is no interaction or communication in any form between these two groups of rats. Intuitively, we know that any trading system, no matter how advanced it may be, degrades in time as more players do the same.

While banks all over the world were imploding and some $50 trillion vanished from global stock markets, the derivatives market grew by an estimated 65 per cent, according to the Bank for International Settlements (BIS). The BIS convenes the world's 57 most powerful central bankers in Basel, Switzerland, for periodic secret meetings. Occasionally, they issue a cry of alarm. In this particular instance, derivatives had soared from $415 trillion at the end of 2006 to $684 trillion in mid-2008. The derivative market is now estimated at $700 trillion (notional or face value, not market value). The world's gross domestic product in 2009 is about $70 trillion and America's is $14 trillion. The total market cap of all major global stock markets is a mere $30 trillion, and the total amount of dollar bills in circulation, most of them abroad, is estimated to be about $830 billion.

Cautious bankers around the world concede that even after listening to experts, they still do not understand derivatives and therefore don't trust them and won't have anything to do with them. And when that weapon of mass destruction explodes, they explain, "Our bank's customers, from all over the world, will be saved from the disaster." George Soros thinks of the current state of the world economy to be in Act two of a three-act play. The meltdown of 2008-2009 was Act One. He believes that entering into a double deep recession is Act Two. Apparently, the total collapse of the economy will be Act Three.

Congress is considering legislation to curb the use of derivatives and other methods that actificially boost returns. One measure proposed by Sen. Blanche Lincoln of Arkansas would bar banks from trading in derivatives. This, in turn, would push almost $300 trillion beyond the reach of regulators. Derivatives would become still more opaque. Some say abolish derivatives trading in the US and push it offshore.

The Greek tragedy over its debt crisis is echoing around the world and certainly in the halls of Congress. Greece's public debt is around 100 per cent of its economy, about the same as for the United States. If you add unfunded US liabilities for social security, Medicare, and Medicaid, the long-term shortfall is $62 trillion, or about the same as the total world GDP, or about $200,000 for each and every American. Fed's current posture is to add liquidity (print money) when markets go down substantially (S/P 500 support at 1040), or stay on the sideline if the mood of the market is positive. Please refer to articles like, Economics 101 . . . , Butterfly Effect . . ., posted at www.nalandainternational.org, for detailed explanation.

When the Dow Jones went into a 1,000-point tailspin and back up in 16 minutes on May 6th of this year, economic and financial prognostication made astrology look respectable. Barron's round table analyst Marc Faber, hedge-fund manager Jim Chanos and Harvard's Kenneth Rogoff told Bloomberg that China's economy will slow and possibly "crash" within a year or two as the nation's property bubble is set to burst. Another Barron's round table analyst Felix Zulauf anticipates the secular bear market bottom should occur at around the market book value. If it happens, then the S/P 500 would have to fall from the current level of about 1100 to the S/P book value of about 500. If I were to consider the forecast of UBS technician Peter Lee, it should happen sometime in 2012. However, in the meantime in coming months, S/P 500 could go over 1,150 depending upon what the Fed does in matters of money supply. Market technicians in general believe the market is in a bullish territory if the index is over 200 days moving average and in bearish territory if it is below the same.

Needless to say that no one can predict the future accurately, unless one happens to be Sahdeva of the Mahabharata, or Cassandra of Greek mythology.

June 2010

Gazing Into the Crystal Ball for 2010

GERALD Celente, who predicted the crash of 2008 and 2009, publishes a trend research report for his clients. Here are his predictions and probable future trends: The stock market will crash again in the later part of 2010. Printing trillions of dollars that don't have real value in the end won't be helpful. Central banks of Western countries have been loaning commercial banks money at an interest rate of zero in exchange for their worthless mortgage-backed securities. Banks in turn buy secured government bonds instead of lending to cash-starved small businesses. 2010 will see the exhaustion of stimulus money, causing the market to crash and sending reverberations all over the world. The Federal Deposit Insurance Company (FDIC) is broke. They're relying on three year's worth of insurance premiums from banks just to stay alive. As central banks keep printing more money, currencies will get clobbered; the winner will be precious metals.

Neosurvivalism: Today's Darwinian survivors are average people making intelligent decisions to prepare for the worst. We must be self-sustaining, doing our best to make it on our own. A commitment to neighbours and community will be the only way for everyone to survive, as we need to help each other get through this crisis. The human population was about one billion a century ago. Our population has increased by about 5 billion people. Naturally, there aren't enough jobs to go around, and as supplies deplete, the welcoming attitude for immigrants that had existed before will deplete as well.

More and more countries are going to focus on kicking out illegal immigrants in the struggle for resources.

TB (Too Big) or not TB: Right now, 34% of the adults in the US are considered obese, and in a mere eight years it is expected to reach 40%. Jobless people of the 2010 depression have much bigger waistlines than those of the 1930 depression. The business of shaping people up will grow with America's waistlines, and even the government will get involved. A trend toward elegance will emerge as people strive to compete for jobs. Everyone is trying to look their best and do their best. Quality counts. Art, architecture, and elegance will get more prominence to lift up the depressed spirit. Bigger is not better in fashion, food, and entertainment. If two candidates for a job are on the same level but one is obese, no matter how unjust one might find it to be, the employer has enough to worry about without considering the higher health insurance cost and taxes due to obesity. I would add that TB has become a health care issue when they discover that the smaller people of Kerala, India, are healthier than the big people of Washington D.C.

Innovation: Celente claims that we can expect our own people's minds to go into high gear in the rough times. He predicts that technology will reach out to the lower socio-economic strata. Making the best with the Least is becoming the new goal. I would suggest if we look east, we see cheaper creations of the highest technology inspired by India's $2200 Nano car and $70 refrigerator. Contrary to popular belief, this is not merely a green movement, but a smart one, and the US could be at the forefront of it.

Not Made In China: As was previously stated, people are going to have to realise how important it is to support one's community and neighbours to live a higher standard of life. Even now we can see the influx of farmer's markets and the resurgence in popularity of the "mom and pop shop."

Celente says "China will become a great pariah as they undercut even the poorest of nations with their products. And so, barriers of trade protectionism will shoot up, which many may think will hurt the economy, but it's a fallacy. Expect to see more "Made in YOUR COUNTRY" products as long as small manufacturers can market their products well."

New Communication Technologies Over Old News: What with the investigative journalism scandals and lack of real news (as opposed to celebrity gossip), people have begun to look elsewhere for the truth. Celente says that "as long as we have net neutrality," NBC, CBS, and other similar networks will either go under or "go web-only." People are beginning to see that they need to take care of themselves and know the truth so as to survive.

Is It Written In The Stars? — Arch Crawford bases most of his projections through the use of astrology. Crawford sees not just another crash this year but dramatic societal changes to go with it. In his words, "We will do everything but guarantee you that stocks will crash worldwide within three months of August 1st (that is between May 1 and November 1). It is expected that technical market analysis of data generated by current market action will assist in pinpointing most danger/opportunity as critical moments approach. The fate of the world is in the balance!" While we don't know Crawford's track record, we, too are concerned about societal strains produced by the strident populist posturing in Washington and elsewhere. We also think this could be a year of food shortages which will strain the lower strata of society. There could be an unusual second quarter that needs to be watched carefully. Institutions, with the backing of the government, have been able to manage markets so far after the March 2009 crash. They can do so **indefinitely** as long as they have a control over the reserve currency, the dollar.

Yes, with their power of printing money they can prevent a crash and manage the market movement within an acceptable band. There is nothing I see out there that would make me change my view about the precious metals market. Banks and governments only have one choice: "Inflate or die!" Or even "Inflate and die" if they lose control walking on the razor's edge. Any move to withdraw liquidity from the market by increasing interest rates would kill the equity marks stone cold dead in a heartbeat. This is a lose-lose situation for the banks and the government, of their own making. On one side of the fence is death by hyper-inflation . . . and on the other hand is death by deflation. Banks and governments have always preferred the inflationary side . . . except for former Fed chairman Paul Volcker who raised rates and killed inflation back in the early 1980s, and saved the dollar in the process . . . But this isn't the 1980s . . . and that option seems unlikely. The last nine years in a row have been 'up' years for precious metals in US dollar terms . . . and, considering the current situation, chances are 2010 should also be an up year. However there is a significant probability that governments could lose control over the economy due to some unexpected, unforeseen Black Swan event like a 9/11 attack. They still are not able to bring unemployment under control.

Barron's editorial (01/18/2010) refers to research funded by the MacArthur Foundation, and deliberated by 21 experts on US fiscal policies for two years. The final outcome is the publication of the book titled, *Choosing the Nation's Fiscal Future*, also available on the website www.nap.org. The conclusion is essentially the same as in the article I wrote, "Sweat Think, and Philosophize", dated September 2008 and posted on www.nalandainternational.org. With the increasing debt load due to the expanded health care and social security programmes vastly more burdensome than the debt for World War II — the more likely outcome could be wild inflation, or being forced to borrow in another currency at a much higher interest rate. So in matters of investment, one needs to be cautious, nimble, and agile. It is indeed a good idea to store essential commodities. In an inflationary climate, it would become difficult to buy them since they become unavailable quickly. Maybe your own intuition, dear friend, could help you propel through this crisis the country is going through.

June 2010

Mutually Assured Financial Destruction

MUTUALLY assured destruction (MAD) is a doctrine of military strategy and national security policy in which a full-scale use of nuclear weapons by two opposing sides would effectively result in the destruction of both the attacker and the defender. The doctrine assumes that each side has enough nuclear weaponry to destroy the other side and that either side, if attacked for any reason by the other, would retaliate with equal or greater force. The expected result is an immediate escalation resulting in both combatants' total and assured destruction. It is now generally hypothesised that the nuclear fallout or nuclear winter resulting from a large-scale nuclear war would bring about worldwide devastation, though this was not a critical assumption to the theory of MAD. The primary application of this doctrine started during the Cold War (1940s to 1990s) in which MAD was seen as helping to prevent any direct full-scale conflicts between the United States and the Soviet Union while they engaged in smaller proxy wars around the world. It was also responsible for the arms race, as both nations struggled to keep nuclear parity, or at least retain second-strike capability. (From Wikipedia)

While we have overcome the Cold War, we are quickly descending into MAD in the financial markets among developed countries, with assured free market destruction as we know it, and with "debt bombs" countering with more printing paper money. However, there are differences in the two situations. First and foremost a nuclear holocaust did not happen, while today, in the views of many market analysts, we are on the path of eventual financial destruction. Unlike the bipolar world of MAD, our interactions are in a globalised world with multiple players making the situation much more complicated. First, the debt bomb went off in America in late 2008, causing tremors all over the world. So the Fed dropped the paper money bomb in a form of a trillion-dollar stimulus package, in essence creating the fiat money and degrading the value of the dollar. That was the beginning of state capitalism replacing free market capitalism after the latter's demise, taking over failed banks, automobile companies, and mortgage companies.

Capitalism takes many forms but all of them can be distinguished by their use of wealth to create more wealth, a broad enough definition to capture both free-market and state capitalism. In the free-market form of capitalism, the job of the state is to "enable" wealth generation by enforcing contracts and limiting the influence of moral vices such as greed — the latter can lead to market failures, which have occurred periodically since the Dutch tulip craze of 1637. Free-market governments attempt to ensure that the economic game is played fairly. In contrast to free-market capitalism, the economy in state-capitalist regimes, like in China and Russia, is dominated by the state agenda. If forced to choose between the protection of the rights of the individual, economic productivity, and the principle of consumer choice, on the one hand, and the achievement of political goals, on the other, state capitalists will choose the latter every time. Continuing the sports game analogy, state capitalists control the referees as well as the main players. (Refer to *The End of the Free Market* by Ian Bremmer)

A few weeks ago Jean-Claude Trichet, the head of the European Central Bank (ECB), was telling the world there was no way the ECB would go nuclear to resolve the Greek debt problem. Then, over the weekend, they went nuclear, creating a trillion dollars out of thin air. Rather than dropping an atomic bomb, however, Europe dropped a money bomb on the markets — a rescue package worth about a trillion dollars. The package included the authority for the ECB to wade into the markets and directly purchase debt. There is perhaps just one thing left to do: *Destroy the euro*. Jean-Claude Trichet, the head of the ECB, should swallow hard . . . admit his failure . . . and print like a madman, devaluing the currency in order to "monetise" the vulnerable Eurozone countries' debts. The euro was *always* a lousy idea — a hodge-podge of dissimilar cultures and economies, stitched together in a "Mad Doctor's" dispensary. The same monetary policy for various and varied economies in the euro zone has created huge imbalances and stress. One medicine cannot cure all the ills.

While Germany has maintained discipline in its financial dealings since the inception of the European Monetary Union, Greece, Italy and Spain have partied. Enjoying the advantage of lower interest and inflation rates, Southern Europeans were caught up in a big credit-driven boom that has gone bust just as it had happened in the US The big bailout, unprecedented in size for Europe, in truth is a bailout of the European banks which were on the hook as the main creditors. The ECB, by following the US in matters of keeping a loose monetary policy, has demolished its own credibility. Apparently the outcome for the euro, dollar and the British pound should be an eventual self-destruction. In the words of Alan Abelson of *Barron's* magazine, "all the central banks in Europe and USA are determinedly printing money like mad to save the world". These actions of money-printing are certainly bullish for gold and silver in the long run. Please note that nothing goes up or down in straight line. Gold is over-bought and should correct itself downwards. There is a huge short position on the euro and could go up for a few months when the shorts are being covered.

State capitalism is very much involved in market manipulation as we are experiencing in the US Institutions, with the blessings of the government, use derivatives to artificially maintain a strong dollar so that the interest rate and therefore the cost of borrowing is maintained at a much lower level. In spite of this effort, the government seems to be losing control over the price of gold. During the September 2008 meltdown, the dollar and US treasury went up over 10% while the gold price was down by 20%. However, gold has outperformed both the dollar and the S&P 500 in each and every time interval of 30 days, 3 months, 6 months, 12 months, 2 years and 5 years. As a matter of fact, gold has gone up by about 170% while the S&P 500 is down by 5% in the last five year time interval (as of May 19th, 2010).

Please note that 70% of the trading volume comes from both foreign and domestic institutions employing their proprietary software. The message here is that the foreign central banks are accumulating gold to strengthen their currencies because their confidence in Western currencies is receding. The great games, played by world powers, are first played in the economic realm before they consider going to war.

Looking at the state of the market, there were two meltdowns in the last 25 days. One of them was an almost death experience. Only the dollar and the gold have been holding well. For graduating students, the toughest test is getting a job. About 80% of 2009 fresh graduates moved back home with their parents, compared to 75% in 2008, and 65%

in 2006. In the view of this writer, the most important responsibility of the executive branch of the government is to keep the jobseekers, and certainly fresh graduates, employed.

May 2010

The Butterfly Effect
Seeds of the Meltdown

In the last two decades, we have experienced the bursting of two bubbles — the first in technology in 2000 and the second in housing in 2008. When exactly were the seeds planted for the current American suffering, with close to 20% combined unemployment and underemployment? Even those who are employed do not feel quite comfortable about their job security. Unemployment is much higher for those fresh graduates coming out of schools and universities. Senior citizens living on fixed income are suffering because the interest and dividend income on their savings and IRA funds have shrunk drastically. The purchasing power of the dollar has been steadily declining, causing increasing hardship to those who exist on meagre income. The average household net worth has shrunk because of the depressed home prices.

The butterfly effect is a metaphor that encapsulates the concept of sensitive dependence on initial conditions in chaos theory; namely, that small changes in the initial condition of a dynamic system may produce large variations in the long-term behaviour of the system. Chaos theory is a field of study in mathematics, physics, and philosophy concerning the behaviour of dynamic systems that are highly sensitive to initial conditions. Here the dynamic system is the American economy, and we are trying to explore and determine what seeds were planted that caused the 2008-2009 chaotic meltdown and a deep recession. Simply stated, the fluttering of butterfly wings in Spain causes a hurricane in Florida.

Some would say that these seeds were planted in the 1980s and '90s with financial deregulation. Some would say that it was due to the Fed's easy monetary policy designed to stimulate economic growth by lowering short-term interest rates and making money less expensive to borrow. I would argue that the seeds were first planted in the 1970s and later reinforced in the 1990s when the market regulations were either removed or not implemented properly.

During the 1992 Presidential election, Ross Perot's role as a third party candidate caused George H.W. Bush to lose to Bill Clinton. Bush lost the election for two reasons — high unemployment and high interest rates. Fed Chairman Alan Greenspan raised interest rates to tighten the money supply to bring some economic discipline whereby good businesses would survive and bad businesses would fail. In a free-enterprise capitalist system, economic cycles are natural. It allows the "dead wood", that is, poorly run businesses, to die while the strong, more efficient businesses survive. The conservative vote got divided between Bush and Perot, giving the presidency to Clinton. There was some validity to Ross Perot's argument in relation to NAFTA (North American Free Trade Agreement). Perot had argued that NAFTA would cause the loss of jobs without sufficient control, as cheap labour became more available from south of the border.

It was during the late 1990s when the CFTC (commodity futures and trading commission) chairperson, Brooksley Born, had proposed to regulate the exploding and out-of-control derivative market. However, she had hit the stonewall erected by then Fed chairman Greenspan and treasury secretary Robert Rubin, also supported by President Clinton. Under great pressure, she resigned the post. Ever since then, the derivative market of over $500 trillion is the big elephant in the room.

Warren Buffett has described it as a financial instrument of mass destruction. Just to put the size of the elephant in perspective, the yearly GDP of USA is about $14 trillion and the entire world GDP is about $65 trillion, while J.P. Morgan, one too-big-to-fail bank, holds derivatives of about $85 trillion. Derivatives do provide useful function of controlling the price movement of securities, similar to a closed loop feedback system to control the movement of a parameter-like speed of a vehicle. However, there has to have some safety mechanism to insure the system stability.

Going back to 1969, the Nixon administration expanded the war in Vietnam, which led to much greater death and destruction in Indo-China. Due to the excessive spending for the Vietnam War and providing arms and ammunitions to Pakistan, the value of the dollar began receding. Countries holding dollars demanded gold for dollars since the dollar was convertible to gold at a rate of $35 per ounce. Half of the gold reserves stored in Fort Knox, about 9,000 tonnes, were delivered to the holders of dollars. With 9,000 tonnes of gold remaining, Nixon officially removed the gold standard. That action created tremendous inflationary pressure, resulting in gold peaking at over $800 per ounce in 1980. The price of all commodities, most importantly oil, rose to the stratosphere, thus creating the terrible inflation of the 1970s. The Yom Kippur war of 1973 had created an oil cartel that had put additional pressure on inflation. A gradual degradation of auto and steel industries due to the cheaper imports from abroad, accelerating manufacturing job loss, added more misery to the people. (Refer to articles, including, "Dysfunctional Detroit, and Sweat" "Think and Philosophize," at www.nalandainternational.org).

The second misfortune for America was the Watergate scandal that caused the country to go through the long-drawn process of impeachment. Watergate was a political scandal in which a break-in into the Democratic National Committee headquarters resulted in the eventual resignation of Richard Nixon. Recorded conversations in President Nixon's offices revealed his involvement with the break-in along with members of his staff. Before Watergate, the United States government was basically considered "God" in the eyes and minds of most Americans. I recall a few of our American friends considered it sinful to evade paying taxes to the American Treasury. This blatant show of corruption changed the attitude of many Americans and created a pattern of cynicism that still exists today.

Thirdly, Nixon was responsible for opening the floodgate of cheap labour from China. He had a very high admiration for Mao Zedong, the leader of Communist China. Nixon was incredibly anxious to meet him and asked his National Security Adviser Henry Kissinger, to arrange a meeting. Pakistan, being friend of both America and China, helped to arrange the meeting. We do know that India and Pakistan have an existing conflict over Kashmir ever since they became independent in 1947. These conflicts escalated as the people of East Pakistan, now Bangladesh, began to migrate to India en-masse from East Pakistan due to the atrocities committed by the Pakistani army.

West Pakistani elites could not accept a Bangli leader Sheikh Mujibur Rahman, who had won the election, as the prime minister of the whole country. Nixon had provided more arms to Pakistan for its defence. Additional arms helped Pakistan Commit great atrocities through "Operation Searchlight" against the people of East Pakistan, killing as many as 3 million and creating 5 million refugees. These events led to the India-Pakistan war of 1971 and later, to the creation of Bangladesh. Nixon's dislike of India's then Prime Minister Indira Gandhi is well-known. He went as far as sending the US Navy's mighty 7th fleet to the Bay of Bengal to pressure

India and help the Pakistani army to save them from defeat. He even encouraged China to invade India to avoid dismembering Pakistan, but with no success. During the meeting with Mao Zedong, Nixon spoke, "This was the week that changed the world. We will do in the years ahead to build a bridge across 16,000 miles and 22 years of hostilities that have divided us. And what we have said today is that we shall build that bridge." This "friendship" of sorts literally opened up the floodgate of cheap labour as American corporations went overseas to increase their profit. This has been the main cause of the transfer of manufacturing jobs for the last 35 years. Nixon resigned in 1974 before he was impeached by the Congress.

So how does the future look on Wall Street? A UBS technician, Peter Lee, sees a correction of about 10 to 15 per cent in the coming summer months, then a rise of about 40 per cent going into 2012. Then he believes the market should test the March 2009 low of DJI of 7000 before 2012 ends. There are two views on interest rates that may influence the stock market. Goldman Sachs projects the interest rate of a 10-year treasury to remain around 3.75 % going into 2011, while Morgan Stanley projects the interest rate of the same to be around 5.5 %. None of the outcomes seem to be very bullish in the view of the writer. Now that Goldman Sachs has been indicted by SEC, the knowledge of market manipulation has entered into the mainstream, which may foreshadow dark times ahead. Europe is already experiencing dark days and maybe even dark times, thanks to the volcanic irruption and Greek debt problem.

April 2010

All the Emperors with No Clothes

LOOKING carefully at the economic indicators, the current state of the Western (G7) economy appears quite dismal. Led by the Europeans, a competitive devaluation of currencies is wreaking havoc on the economic recovery prospects for the Western nations. The devalued Euro will not help the US and Canada, a tired country with little or no gold reserves to back the Canadian loonies. People delude themselves into thinking that Greece, Spain, U.K., Canada, California, New York and the entire US will solve their problems through a tightening of the fiscal belt. Economists believe that governments should start cutting their spending and increase taxes, but such measures could result in astronomical unemployment as seen in Africa. The G7 apparently is a form of a grand Ponzi scheme, with little or no productive backing, like the defunct Enron. The emperors of the West, just about a century later, are essentially broke by spending their fortune on an unsustainable lifestyle.

As I have opined in earlier articles, governments need to focus on production, not consumption, to create wealth. Paper money becomes money only when it is convertible to an asset class that is acceptable and respected the world over. Unfortunately, governments are not showing any signs that they will be heading in the right direction.

Reviewing the history of currency, the barter system came first and continued for a millennia, but that initial arrangement was replaced by a more efficient and sophisticated system of world currency in the form of precious metals. Europe became rich because of the Industrial Revolution together with colonisation that provided raw materials. The riches and wealth of Europe essentially disappeared by the middle of the 20th century as a result of the two world wars and government socialistic tendencies. Following World War II, America came of age and amassed more than half of the world's gold and built Fort Knox to store it. In the post-WWII era, if you owned the dollar you also owned gold since the dollar was convertible into gold. America, as a victor of WWII, with the support of the Allies, was able to establish the dollar as the world reserve currency. But human nature rarely fails; power corrupts men sooner or later, if not in the first generation then in the second or third. America, though born of idealism, is an unexpected example of how corruption and decadence seep in and spread.

The US soon used its global dominance to print money to finance a military-industrial complex, multiple wars (Korea, Vietnam, Iraq, etc.), to dole out foreign aid, and to exert its political influence all over the world. Some of us would have to confess that we took advantage of the situation since we came to America for higher education, but we took employment in the same military-industrial complex instead of going back to our homelands.

This spending extravaganza eroded the integrity of the US dollar. America maintained the facade for a while by exchanging foreign dollars for gold, with France leading the charge to demand gold for dollars. When half of the gold, about 9,000 metric tonnes, evaporated from Fort Knox in a short span between the late 1960s and the early 1970s, President Nixon disconnected the dollar from gold. That decision marked the end of the true international trading standard. If we compare currencies to the blood of a living organism, the removal of gold as an anchor, or as a "quality controller", caused the decline in the "nutritional" value of currencies. As a result, for the last 40 years, the US and the rest of the world have embarked on a nonstop printing spree. Trillions have been spent on wars, trillions to save the banks, trillions on health care, and trillions for the good life of the chosen few, and the spending spree continues on and on just like the Energizer Bunny in the battery advertisement.

Please note that after the peak was established in the '50s and '60s, the US growth rates of GDP, employment, and income have been declining. For example, the average GDP growth rate peaked in the 1940s at 5.5%, and it has been declining steadily with the lowest in the first decade of the 21st century at 1.9%. (*The Economist* magazine, Feb 27th, p. 36).

Ironically this situation has been brought upon us with the blessings of all the great minds of our era including John Maynard Keynes, many Nobel Laureate economists, and rocket scientists who have applied the laws of natural science to economics, with very little regard for human psychology. The great minds of the Western world that include psychologist Sigmund Freud, political theorist and sociologist Karl Marx, physicist Rene Descartes and economist John Maynard Keynes have all failed in varying degrees.

I submit that two significantly important causes for the decline are the Western belief that nature must serve humanity's interests and the "Holier than Thou" mindset. On the other hand, the Eastern belief states that humanity must have reverence for nature since she is the Mother, and second, the truth is never absolute. Recall the truth described by the parable, "Elephant and the Blind Men". Ultimately, humanity and nature must exist in a symbiotic way. Growth does not have to be at the expense of the environment. Growth can be extended seamlessly from without to within.

With the institutional manipulation in full bloom, the economy and markets give an impression that we have overcome all the excessive indulgence of the past. Oblivious to reality, stock prices are driven up, down or sideways by proprietary computer programmes with devilish cunning to suck money from idealistic dreamers who believe that markets are free and unbiased. When the stock price drops in a split second, the little guy probably feels like Charlie Brown when Lucy tempts him to kick the football, but falls on his behind every season. Faster than the shark attack or a blink of an eye, high frequency trading machines, employed by the great parasitical vampire squid, a.k.a. Goldman Sachs, alertly look for their prey. The name, "vampire squid", coined by Matt Taibbi of *Rolling Stone* magazine, seems most appropriate metaphor for the predatory mentality of the bank. These machines, employed by a few giant banks, can read your order in a microsecond, and squeeze the little guys to their tolerance level for a nickel or a dime, billions of times during every trading day and make millions for their owners. Is it legal? Probably yes, but it is certainly not ethical. Nevertheless, the banks do it to everyone, including to their own clients. The Secretaries of Treasury for the last two decades, Robert Rubin, Henry Paulson, and Timothy Geithner, all came from Goldman Sachs. Wall Street in essence has been able to highjack Washington. Democracy seems to have been replaced by plutocracy. There is a recent news story that Europe, under the leadership of German Chancellor Angela Markel and the French President Nicolas Sarkozy, has declared war on Wall Street by limiting the sales, of some of their derivative products, thanks to Goldman Sachs involvement in helping Greece to hide its debt.

At this stage of economic history, our only solution will be to bring back the discipline that removes the tendency of governments and "Too-Big-to-Fail" corporations to take advantage of others. It is apparent that only the markets, with little but appropriate supervision by policymakers, will determine the next policy system. In some ways, precious metals will be one of the participants if not the only one. In the meantime, we will see uncertainty, volatility and defaults. Keeping substantial cash, investing in precious metals and their mining stocks, and little in growth stocks is a good idea as long as the money supply M3 is stable in an environment of rising mortgage defaults and unemployment. Trading agility is extremely important in this market environment because a black swan could appear at any moment with devastating results. There are a few observers who claim that M3 in reality is manipulated and rising. The real inflation rate given on www.shadowstat.com is significantly higher. Highly respected market analyst Marc Faber advises people to keep buying precious metals at equal time intervals for the rest of their lives, since the money-printing press is being operated at a much higher speed than the mining of precious metals. Well, Indians have been doing it for thousands of years because they have learnt that rulers almost always cheat their subjects by devaluing their currency.

March 2010

Economics 101 and the State of the World Economy

A GOOD image for the state of the world economy is a giant bathtub whose water tap is controlled by the central banks of countries around the world. The water level in the bathtub represents the overall strength of the economy. The banks are keeping the taps open at this time by printing money to stimulate slumping economies. This giant bathtub also has several large unplugged holes through which the water is gushing out uncontrollably. Each hole is created by a mini-explosion due to an economic event like a jump in the mortgage default rate or a rise in the number of unemployed. The world's fundamental economic problems created by banks will not disappear simply by keeping the printing presses running nonstop. One "hole" was created by Greece, which deviated from the Euro-imposed discipline of keeping the government deficit below 3% of GDP, and another was created due to the implosion of the Dubai economy caused by excessive debt. In the USA. the increasing deficit, now over 9% of GDP, due to bail out and stimulus packages, decreasing tax revenue and sagging demand seems to be a perennial hole. When they plug one hole, another is created. Please note that we have not addressed in this image the long-term leaks such as transfer of wealth due to consumption much greater than production.

Central bankers insist on quantitative easing by increasing the money supply or printing money as a short-term solution, which is analogous to pouring water into the bathtub, but at the same time the water is gushing out due to the holes at the bottom. Deflationary pressure, due to the oversupply of goods and services and decreasing employment, also causes the water level in the bathtub to fall. When asset prices keep declining due to the oversupply of goods and services and insufficient demand, the water level falls, thanks to Adam Smith's supreme law of demand and supply. Falling bank lending at the fastest rate in history is another deflationary hole that can be plugged only when the rise in economic growth accelerates. Total bank lending has dropped by about three quarter of a trillion dollars in the last 12 months. The broadest money supply measure, M3, a leading indicator of the state of the economy, has been contracting at a rate of 5.6% over the last three months. The risk of a double-dip recession or even worse is growing by the day.

Economists' perception of the current state of the world economy is divided. Those who look at the top of the bathtub see this as an inflationary situation as they focus on the abundance of paper money in the form of stimulus packages to jump-start the economic engine. Those who dare to look at the bottom of the bathtub recognise the fundamental problems and see uncontrolled deflation in our future. Currently, no one knows for sure what will happen in the future due to the uniqueness of the current state of the economy. In March 2009, the market crashed, and the inflationary pressure since then has been marginal. The water level seems to rise when the taps are opened, and on the surface the markets seem to stabilise. However, when a new crisis arises due to fundamental economic issues, new holes emerge and the water level starts falling once again. European countries like Portugal, Italy, England and Spain, or even troubled states in the US including California, New York and Illinois, also have the same problem: the deficit as a percentage of GDP is far greater than the acceptable level of 3%. Until the underlying inadequacies are addressed, this systematic pattern will continue to plague the world economies.

In the long term, central bankers tend to err on the inflationary side as they had during the 2002-2007 period after the recession of 2000 and the 9/11 event. Economic history has always been on the side of inflation. In fact, 3% inflation rate is the current acceptable level central bankers shoot for. Olivier Blanchard, the IMF's chief economist, now recommends that central bankers should raise their target to 4% inflation rate (*The Economist*, February 20th, 2010 issue). Even staunch ultra free-market economist F.A. Hayek, whose views come from the Austrian school of economics, and are the opposite of those of John Maynard Keynes, a strong proponent of government intervention, agree that when the economy falls off the cliff, the intervention of central bankers in creating more credit and money is essential to a avoid catastrophic depression.

Now more than ever before, all the markets in the world are interconnected. It is indeed a reversal of fortune that the Western countries now prefer that the emerging economies of China, India and Brazil increase their GDP growth rate. The Western countries would like to see stronger emerging market economies that will generate a demand for the export of goods and services from Western countries. Sooner or later, the holes of the bathtub will get plugged and the water level will rise and even overflow, bringing the economy to an inflationary domain. I do hope they get plugged sooner than later.

So how does one invest when the treasury yields are near zero with high stock market volatility? I would prefer a mixed asset allocation that includes short-term (five years and shorter) investment grade bonds, precious metals, substantial cash, and a bit invested in very stable growth stocks. Those who are willing to take some risk can consider shorting US treasury bonds. The logic of short-selling US treasury bonds is very simple. America is drowning in a sea of debt at a near-zero interest rate. Essentially, there is no upside other than the belief in the strength of the dollar. Undoubtedly, there will be inflation at some point in the future. Currently the decreasing money supply M3 shows deflationary pressure. Only when most of the holes of the bathtub are plugged, meaning M3 and employment start rising and the real estate markets are stabilised, will the equity markets perform better. However, if the rate of inflation goes out of control and keeps rising, the long bonds will get slaughtered while precious metals will probably outperform almost all other asset classes. I do emphasise that one needs to be nimble and agile in this highly volatile market.

February 2010

Weakening Dollar in a Civilisation Shift

In ancient times, gold coins circulated far and wide across the globe just as paper currency does today. Even after the birth of paper currency, the gold standard for paper money ensured its stability. Between the Battle Waterloo of 1815 and the Great Depression of the 1930s, the pound sterling ruled, but it was still convertible into gold. Even in the 20th century, from the Depression years to the late 1960s, the dollar could be converted into gold. In fact, Section 19 of this country's founding monetary legislation, the Coinage Act of 1792, prescribed the death penalty for any official who fraudulently debased the people's money. The Act was later repealed because Keynesians opposed it. Today, however, there is no backing for the US dollar except the hollow faith of the US government. The world is rapidly losing respect for the dollar, and our currency now resembles General Motors in that our best days are behind us.

Let us turn our attention to the economic views of Keynes and Mises discussed in my earlier article on the dollar to get a deeper understanding of our current economic problems. The two men represent a pair of opposites in the realm of economics. In a recession, Keynes encouraged government spending to stimulate the economy, while Mises opposed government intervention. Would Keynes be wrong today? In short, yes. Keynes' support of uncontrolled government expenditures would worsen the current situation, although it is occasionally good to have a controlled elastic currency at the government's disposal. The pure paper currency monetary system of Keynes creates "black holes" of secrecy and violent volatility that results in unjust imbalances. As we have shifted drastically in the direction of fiscal recklessness bringing us closer to potential hyperinflation, we need to restore a balance and harmony with a return to sound principles of saving and investment in productive assets. America has consumed more than it has produced since 1976, as measured by the trade balance, which amounts to a deficit of 32 years and counting.

If the rulers of the country keep printing money for their advantage, purchasing power is sure to fall in proportion to the increase in paper currency. If the inflation rate is much higher than the interest rate, purchasing power will keep dwindling. However, if the interest rate is much higher than the inflation rate, the currency is bound to become stronger reminiscent of the 1980s. Money flows to where it is treated the best, where returns are high. Holders of American bonds are being penalised with a negative real return, causing significant capital flowing away from America.

If we look back to the 1980s, Fed chairman Volcker squeezed liquidity out of the system by increasing the interest rate. The dollar became one of the strongest currencies with an inflation-adjusted interest rate topping over 10%, and it remained strong through 2000 with the real interest rate declining gradually to 3.5%. After 9/11, pessimism and fear dominated, creating an economic slowdown. The interest rate dropped close to 0%. With the promise of easy credit, the markets took off in 2003. However, the dollar was becoming ever weaker. In a healthy economy, the deficit as a percentage of GDP should be less than 3%. If it is over 5% of the GDP, the currency is bound to get weaker. Currently the deficit has soared to over 10% of GDP and climbing. The dollar, in terms of gold, has gone down below 30%. America had gone through a situation similar to the 2008 financial tsunami when the stock market crashed in 1929, resulting in depression. Newly elected president Franklin Delano Roosevelt was wise when he didn't remove the dollar pegged to gold. All he did was to inflate the economy only once by lowering the peg to gold from $20/oz to $35/oz. He maintained sufficient discipline to keep a constant purchasing power at $35/oz of gold by maintaining gold as an anchor.

In our time of astronomical deficits, the government issues debt paper to finance the deficits. The first stage of the money-printing cycle is that investors keep buying. When the buyers realise the risk associated with the excessive borrowing, they curtail their purchase of the government paper. The next stage is that the government buys their own paper, also known as "quantitative easing", or I would call "legalised counterfeiting". As the deficit keeps increasing with more and more paper currency printed, the rest of the world realises the problem, and that is the start of runaway inflation. During the hyperinflation of the 1980s in Brazil, people would keep the currency in hand for the shortest possible period, spending it in the same hour they received it. They knew that the next hour the price of essential goods would be higher.

The US is in the middle of a perfect storm that will have significant ripple effects throughout the world. Currently the unemployment in US is in double digits, and some estimate true unemployment, including underemployment, at close to 20%. Bank problems are still not resolved, and those issues will also cause more printing of money. The toxic debt issue still looms large. A huge portion of the derivative market, about $500 trillion, is worthless. So far over 100 US banks have failed. The FDIC has run out of money. There is a good chance that more than one major bank will fail. For example, J.P. Morgan holds over $100 billions in derivatives, and if and when those collapse, JPM could face a philosophical death.

All of these issues will continue to weaken the dollar over time. These problems are bound to proliferate worldwide.

There is a significant probability that the world financial system as we know it may not survive, and it will have to be revived in a different form. Money printing keeps rulers in power for a while, but ultimately they are thrown out because they destroy the economy. Voltaire had said in 1729 that paper money will eventually return to its intrinsic value — zero. The people have been put in these dire straits by their politicians, and it could take many years to come out of it. As Einstein wisely commented, "don't expect the people who caused a problem to solve it." Matt Taibbi, in the December issue of *Rolling Stone* magazine, narrates the story of how President elect Obama brought in the same gang of Wall Street who created the financial tsunami of 2008.

Is the world following India in matters of savings and social security? China is certainly doing it, encouraging their citizens to put their savings in gold and silver. People in the Western countries are doing the same by buying the gold and silver coins. Gold and silver in India represents their IRA and Keogh, the savings for a rainy day, the dowry for a daughter's wedding, and more. We are shifting from a dollar hegemony to the age-old 5000-year-old system of saving in the form of gold, silver and other tangible assets. We know that John Paulson, Jim Rogers and many more all over the world, the billionaire fund managers, are making a big bet on gold, silver and other resources. Petroleum exporting Arab countries plan to float their own currency calling it "Gulfo" and modelled after the Euro, some time next year, probably backed by the gold reserve.

Ambrose Evans-Pritchard of *The London Telegraph* narrates the story about the rising economic powers of Asia and the Middle East. They have lost confidence in Western currencies and are replacing them gradually with gold. Currently, on average, these countries have only about 2.2% of their foreign reserve compared to over 35% for the G-7. They would have to buy about $700 billion worth of gold to have half (18%) of their foreign reserve at the current price. The top Chinese banker Zhu Min indicated that they buy gold when the price goes to some support level. The implication here is that the gold price may drop some but cannot crash. The rise of the gold price does not seem to be due to the momentum players. Perhaps it is a civilisation shift. I would call this reversing the direction of the pendulum, the "laws of karma" at work – transfer of wealth from West to East! Please note that India was one of the richest countries at the end of the 17th century before Robert Clive from England arrived in India. I would urge you, dear friend, to review the first article on the dollar (Nov 21, 2009), posted on www.nalandainternational.org to get a deeper understanding of current economic matters.

January 2010

Dollar
Past, Present and Future

I BOUGHT my first mid-size car for about $3,000 in 1961. A similar car would cost about $30,000 today. On the surface, it seems that in the last 50 years the value of a dollar has dwindled to a dime. Even more disturbing is the UCLA tuition fees. Today it is over $8,000 per year, compared to about $200 I paid in 1960. I do need to know what the future holds for the dollar. Is it a case of history repeating itself, with the dollar associating itself with God and gold in the future? We need to review the past to gaze into the future, when the dollar with its inscription, "In God we trust" was tied to gold.

The word "dollar" is historically related to the Bohemian tolar (16th century) and much later to the Slovenian tolar (1991), the daalder in the Netherlands, and the daler in Sweden, Denmark, and Norway. Initially the American dollar was pegged to about 1.3 ounces of fine silver and later on, it was pegged to gold at about $20 per ounce of pure gold. President Roosevelt, during the Depression years, devalued the dollar by changing the ratio to $35 per ounce.

At the end of World War II, treaties were signed in order to establish a common currency to be used among nations. In his article, *It's Time to End World War II*, Hugo Salinas Price, the founder of Mexico's *Electra* retail chain, pronounces that the essential agreement is "one that established that gold should be the money to be used to settle all trade deficits between nations, but in lieu of gold, dollars could be used to settle these deficits. In forcing on the Breton Woods Agreements the acceptance of the dollar as a means of settling international debts, along with gold, the US established the will of a victorious power to continue to plunder the whole world." General de Gaulle (President of France, 1959-1969) has been quoted as saying that this was "an exorbitant and unnecessary privilege" given to America. And so, it was indeed a privilege of the victor in World War II. The perception that America took advantage after WW II has acquired more credence in a recently published book by Dussmann Kulturfaufhaus in Germany. The book has created uproar among Germans because it claims that Germany gave away its sovereignty by signing an agreement that granted undue advantage to the US It also claims that all German gold, even now, is being held in the US

The favoured status of American currency eventually led to leverage in paying for imports and the accumulation of huge trade deficits. The victor, expanding its money supply with little discipline, became the largest debtor country in the history of the world. In Hugo's words, "the exporting countries, not being nuclear powers, were afraid to demand gold in payment of their export surpluses, since such a request would very probably irritate the great power." When countries like France asked for gold and not dollars, President Nixon removed the dollar linkage with gold, making the dollar a fiat currency. By running a huge trade deficit which arose out of its expansion of credit and consequent money-printing, the US was able to send abroad masses of dollars to pay for imports. The exporting countries received dollars — not gold — for their export surpluses to the US The dollars began to pile up in foreign central banks as "reserves".

Commerce is an eminently peaceful activity. The seller forces no one to buy; the buyer forces no one to sell. The means of payment in commerce, since written history began, has been either goods for goods, i.e., barter, or goods for gold or silver — a perfected form of barter. But anything else, any innovation, anything *decreed* to be a means of payment by anybody whatsoever, cannot be anything but an imposition, a violation of the rules of commerce.

The present ruinous condition of the world's finances and its lopsided industrial development has not yet corrected itself. If anything, we are in the "eye of the hurricane" for the moment. Over the course of the past few years, the dollar has continually spiralled downward. The dollar, as a *Paper Atlas,* is subjected to hold the weight of the world on its weakening shoulders. Currently, the devaluing dollar has to uphold its strength as the world currency if it wants to prevent the potential to end abruptly and violently. Few observers believe that the dollar may gain some strength for a short while. The world has gone short on dollars in a very big way. A few examples include investors sending funds abroad to purchase emerging market assets, the issuance of dollar-denominated bonds, not in their own currencies by sovereign nations, and going out of Europe's way to borrow greenbacks instead of the Euro. So the odds are increasing that the dollar may rise in the near future once the momentum reverses, causing short sellers to cover their shorts.

So what does this once-powerful dollar have in store for its future? Hugo Price believes that "the world's principal powers should convene and come to an agreement for the establishment of the world's monetary and financial systems," where he deems the basis of gold, even silver, to exemplify "a neutral, real and objective medium for commerce and finance." Even though the world's reserve currency seldom changes, the slowing US economy and the devaluation of the dollar may cause an alternative currency to come into play. US policymakers claim that a declining dollar will help American exporters to export more. However, other countries, particularly those with their currencies tied to the dollar, seem to be doing the same, maintaining a very low interest rate. Competing currency devaluation by the central bankers seems to be a fool's race to the bottom. Recall that the currency is the lifeblood of an economy, and making it weaker is certainly not healthy.

The current purchase of some 200 tonnes of gold by the Reserve Bank of India has caused the dollar to weaken further. For the first time, a major central bank of a significantly large economy is buying gold, reversing the trend of last several decades when central banks usually sold gold. Before India's purchase of gold, the jewellery market used 80% of the total gold supply, with all other markets, mostly technology, taking in the remaining 20%. Today the financial segment, that includes hoarding by central banks and investors, has a 50% share of the gold supply. It seems we are going "Back to the Future" (Recall the movie starring Michael Fox), as it has been in the past before the 1950s when world trade transactions were settled bartering for goods or exchanging with gold and silver. Officially the US central bank holds over 8,000 metric tonnes, the largest among all central banks. However, only the Fed and bullion banks know how much is left after leasing and short-selling to keep the dollar strong. In comparison, the Reserve Bank of India currently holds much less than a thousand tonnes, but Indian citizens hold over 20,000 tonnes. Almost 100 years ago, **John Maynard Keynes** chided India for its "ruinous" love of the "barbaric relic". Perhaps central banks were reading their Keynes over the last two decades, during which anti-gold sentiment pervaded. It seems that Indian experience is winning over those who thought they can control nature in general and the human psyche in particular. Another economist from Austria mostly ignored by Keynesians, **Ludwig von Mises**, had contradicted Keynes' view and probably learnt from Indian experience about the greed of rulers that makes them cheat their subjects by weakening the currencies they control.

Pierre Lassonde, CEO of *Franco Nevada*, believes that the gold price should rise at a level when the ratio of Dow Jones index to the price of gold goes below 2. Currently the ratio is a little over 9. This ratio has gone twice to about one in 1934, when the Dow and the gold price were about 35, and in 1980 when they were about 800. Aaron Regent, president of the largest producer of gold, *Barrick Gold*, believes that we passed the peak production of gold sometime in 2000. The ore grades have fallen from 12 grams in the 1950s to about 3 grams per tonne recently and the trend has never reversed, adding more pressure to the gold price. I have recommended buying gold as an insurance against the ravages of inflation in this newspaper first in 2002 when gold was trading a little over $300. The bullish case for gold could go for another five years based upon cycle studies, and the price could go over $2,000.

November 2009

Irrational Optimism

As a young nation, America has always preferred to boldly look ahead to a limitless future without much consideration for the past. Because we have such a brief history, we tend to cut ties with past events as a matter of course. In one regard, this perspective grants Americans the freedom to quickly overcome calamities with optimism and courage. However, when held unchecked, our short-term memory has clouded our judgement and created an irrational optimism borne out of a refusal to learn from past misfortune. This recession has its roots in our willful ignorance of all the warning signs related to loose credit, shaky loans, and exotic financial instruments. Apparently we stand at a precarious point in our economic crisis, and we need to finally face facts rather than dwell in a fantasy world of our own invention. The recession will not evaporate just because the politicians and the public feel that Americans have endured enough pain and suffering. On the contrary, as the economic indicators worsen, we may very well be just getting started with our downward slide. If we are to learn one lesson from the financial collapse of 2008, it is that America needs to balance its unbridled optimism with some humility and a desire to avoid past mistakes.

When we examine the various key economic indicators, we see a consistency in the dismal nature of the numbers. National unemployment is now at 9.8%, the highest it has reached since 1983. More than 90% of American financial institutions are technically insolvent. So far this year, 95 banks have failed and counting. The number of US lenders unable to collect over 20% of their loans has hit an 18-year high. The collective net worth of the Forbes 400, America's richest group, has fallen by $300 billion in the last year, a drop of almost 20%. As residential foreclosure rates continue to rise, banks are holding their breath in anticipation of the wave of 5-year interest-only commercial mortgages that will be due in the next one to three years. When the commercial real estate foreclosure onslaught begins, banks may face a second financial crisis. Consumer confidence has dipped, creating a bad omen for retailers as they look ahead to the all-important holiday season. As small and mid-size businesses lack capital for expansion, the unemployment rate will inevitably rise well into the double digits.

Bill Gross, the manager of the largest bond fund, and feature columnist Allen Abelson of Barron's believe that the US government needs to be more concerned about deflation than inflation, contradicting what the stock market is telling us. Usually the message from the bond market is more accurate than the same from the stock market. The implication here is that interest rates should remain low for years to come. Highly credible monetary experts believe that America has no choice but plan an orderly decline of the dollar to 50% in ten years to get out of the deflationary spiral and the huge deficit. The implication here is that America needs to introduce about 7% inflation every year for the next ten years. Mark Faber, a prophet of gloom and doom and a Barron's round table contributor, believes that the dollar could sink in value very rapidly. His very recent statement was that "it took 100 years for the dollar to go down to a dime, but the dollar of today could go down to a dime in less than 15 years".

Only recently, there was a news story, denied by the Arabs, that they are secretly negotiating with China, Russia, Brazil and France to trade oil in a basket of currencies replacing the dollar. If it is true, the downward spiral of the dollar could accelerate. The great game the big powers play is always to gain advantage over any other trading partner. It is apparent that America is losing its leverage in the world currency market based upon the statements in the news media.

Ambrose Evans Pritchard of the *London Telegraph*: "You can date the end of dollar hegemony from China's decision last month to sell its first batch of sovereign bonds in Chinese yuan to foreigners. It is this shift in Asia and Latin America that threatens dollar domination, not just the pricing of oil contracts".

Fund manager Vitaly Nesis: "Domination of the dollar as the world currency has started to decline and gold will be its natural descendent. Gold should stay in the driving seat despite the spin coming from G-7 bankers. Perceived recovery is probably a mirage communicated by gullible media".

Chinese government banker: "Transitional currency in the move away from dollar may well be gold". The golden rule over the ages has been that "those who own the most gold rule the world".

Dow Theory letter editor, Richard Russell: "Meanwhile, a great bull market starts . . . a bull market that mirrors the demise of the dollar. Gold is priced in dollars, and as the dollar weakens, it takes an increasing amount of fiat dollars to buy an ounce of gold. Beginning in 1999, gold started up in a primary bull market. In my personal opinion, this is fated to be one of the greatest bull markets in history. It will be a bull market built on not one, but two powerful human emotions — both greed and fear. The speculative third phase lies ahead. Slowly but surely, the US public will finally realise that the US government is bankrupt both morally and monetarily. People will panic into gold. . . . I believe that there will be a world panic to buy gold. This will set off one of the wildest and most explosive bull markets in history".

America once owned the most gold held in Fort Knox. Today, we do not know how much gold America has since it is kept secret. Congressman Ron Paul's request to audit for gold reserve has been vehemently opposed by the Fed. On 10/08/2009, gold traded at $1055, the highest level ever in its trading history.

October 2009

Die-Hard Illusions

WE are in an age of bubble markets. Bubbles create both a highly overpriced and also a deflated class of assets at the same time. These formations are not new; in fact, the boom and bust of the Panama Canal and the rail-road are great examples of such occurrences. In the past, there was a long period of moderated asset prices between bubbles, but this is not so nowadays. We had two bubble formations back to back in a short period of 16 years, thanks to former Federal Reserve (Fed) chairman Alan Greenspan (*Maestro Greenspan, the Black Swan*, by N. Doshi). The technology bubble occurred from 1992 to 2000 while the commodities were going through deflation. During the housing bubble which between 2001 and 2007, almost all classes of assets were going up in price. The current Fed chairman, Ben Bernanke, is pumping money into the system that could help generate the third set of bubbles. Bubbles make most investors feel rich, but only for a short time. Once the bubble bursts, investors feel poorer. Bubbles are a form of illusion, far away from reality.

Our Eastern traditions proclaim that our awakened state of mind is an illusion compared to the fourth (Turiya, selfless and desire-less) state, just as the dream state is an illusion compared to the awakened state. However, even in an awakened state of mind, we cannot escape Einstein's relativity due to our existence in nature — nature creates a multi-dimensional space bounded by pairs of opposites. Our existence, individually as well as socially, in this space is not static but changing. Not only do we move in this space, but so do the boundaries move. Currently, the economic space is shrinking. Our response as people should be to correct this so that we move closer to the centre to reach balance and harmony. This correction is not to overspend, but to save. However, our government's response does not seem to be appropriate — in fact, it keeps increasing the spending in matters of energy (flawed and protectionist carbon cap & trade bill) and health care. The government gave away $4,500 for each older car that was turned in to help the auto industry get on its feet, but in the process, billions of tax payers' dollars will be spent. As I understand it, they have been junking these old cars instead of exporting them to countries in which they can be used. Those who are taking the advantage now will not buy another car in year 2010 or 2011. The implication here is that we have pushed the problem to next year or the year after.

Based upon centuries of human experience, we know that the free market does the job much more efficiently than the government bureaucrats. Even though we are letting the government do the job, we know that our problem is with leverage, extreme borrowing and spending. Even so, government experts believe they can overcome the problem by borrowing or printing trillions more. Vice President Joe Biden said on CNN, "We have to spend money to keep from going bankrupt". As of now around the first week of August 2009, they have about $12 trillion committed to one form or another. Adjusted for inflation, that's more than twice the entire amount of money spent during WWII. The government is fighting deflationary forces tooth and nail by more credit and consumption, rather than accepting a painful adjustment period (as it so happened in the early 1980s). This process adapted by the government is putting the entire nation at a great risk. As the private sector continues to pay back debt, the government printing money may not result in immediate inflation. However, over a period of time, all these unnecessary bailouts are going to cause a massive inflation.

In Economics 101 we learn that prices are determined by supply and demand. What is not usually taught in schools, however, is that the "price" — i.e. the purchasing power — of money is also established by these same two economic determinants. Economists focus quite extensively on the supply of money, which is the total quantity of dollars in circulation. The demand for money, however, is largely ignored. The demand should grow close to one and a quarter per cent per year, since that is the growth rate of the population in the US. However, John Williams (www.shadowstats.com) estimates that based upon M3, the broadest measure of money supply, we have is about $15 trillion in circulation. That comes out to be about $50,000 for every American assuming the country's population is 300 million. The money in circulation 100 years ago was about 200 dollars for every American. The growth rate of money on average in the last 100 years has been about 6 per cent per year. However, the growth rate of M1, tl money supply reported by Fed that includes currency anu bank deposits, in the last 12 months alone is estimated to be over 18%. So where has that money gone?

A good portion of the TARP money is used to strengthen the banks' balance sheet and lift up the stock market. It has not yet significantly trickled down to the lower levels. However, the insiders, meaning the high level officers and owners of corporations, are selling heavily booking profit. But some market experts preach not to fight the tape and the Fed, implying to be a trend follower, and remain invested in the market, as long as the Fed keeps interest rates low. I would argue to be invested in markets of your choice only if you are agile, patient with strong guts, and have deep pockets. Rationally, it is good to buy at the bottom, but in reality it is much more difficult to catch the lowest of the low.

On August 7th, the Fed reported that consumer credit fell a whopping 10.3 billion dollars. That was far steeper than estimates. Revolving debt (mostly credit cards) fell over 5 billion dollars. This was the tenth month in a row that credit card debt fell (an all-time record string). The drop in consumer credit is not good for the economy, since the US consumer is traditionally 70% of the economy. The implication here is that the recovery may not be self-sustaining; it could drop again double dipping like the "W".

August 2009

A Tale of Two Metals
Gold and Silver

JUST as in the novel, *A Tale of two Cities,* written by Charles Dickens, about London and Paris during French revolution and the unflattering social parallels, this is an article about gold and silver. The poor man's symbol of wealth, silver, has been treated unfairly by design or otherwise by institutions with the blessings of governments.

I have written extensively on gold (three articles at www.nalandainternational.org), but the story of silver is equally compelling, if not more so. Gold and silver have been used as money for thousands of years, for their beauty, rarity and being chemically unchanging and stable. The name silver, probably for its beautiful lustre, also happens to be the name of a currency of India, the rupee (Devanagari: Rupyak), since the dawn of human civilisation. Few are aware of the gradual disappearance of existing silver in the world, and even fewer people are aware of the resulting inevitable increase in silver's value.

For about a hundred years, from 1792-1891, money was pegged to both metals, gold at about $20.7 per ounce, and silver at $1.3 per ounce in America. So the ratio of the price of gold to that of silver (PR) remained 16. During Queen Victoria's time, the British Government had the pound sterling in England and the rupee in India pegged to an equal weight of gold and silver, keeping the PR at about 15, and maintaining 15 rupees for every pound sterling. An old timer, like this writer, would recall that there were 20 shillings to a pound, 12 pence to a shilling, and 16 annas to a rupee. So the British had one anna equal to one pence during their rule over India.

However, there were international trade problems associated with the bi-metal monitory standard. One of the problems observed by the British economist, John Maynard Keynes, was the deflationary danger since traditionally India was literally a "sink" of gold and silver. Even today, Indians hold a portion of their wealth in gold and silver. It was Indian hoarding that triggered Keynes's mind discovering the relationship between savings and investment which culminated in his *General Theory of Employment, Interest, and Money*. To quote author Glyn Davies in his book, *History of Money* . . ., "Keynes learnt a lot from India, and the world learnt a lot from Keynes." He advocated making currency elastic by removing the gold standard, essentially in order to control unemployment.

When silver was unpegged from the dollar after 1934, PR had gone up to about 35 on average fluctuating from 30 to as high as 65, after F.D.R. had devalued the dollar pegging at $35 per ounce of gold. When Nixon removed the gold standard alltogether, both gold and silver started to go up, gold peaking at about $800 and silver at $50 per ounce during 1979-80. The range of PR was about 15 to 38, with an average of about 34. From 1981 to 2002, commodities including precious metals were in a bear market, first, due to keeping very high interest rates under Paul Volcker as Fed chairman, then under Greenspan as the chairman. The price of silver, silver being a very small market compared with other markets, was easy to keep suppressed by selling "paper" short, meaning the shorts were only entries in a computer. Options in the commodity market are paper entries, deliveries are usually not made to the purchasers. Bullion banks, with the blessings of the Fed and Treasury, do the paper short of both, gold and silver, to keep the perception of inflation in control. PR during this time period, was fluctuating in the range of low 50s' to high 90s'. The bull market of commodities got initiated after 2002 due to a high demand from Asia, and bullion banks could not keep the lid on the price of gold and silver. PR has been in the range of 50 to 70 in this time period, and currently close to 68, (August 21st, 2009, gold @ $950, silver @ $14).

There are three possible forces that could propel the price of silver to go exponentially upward. The first one could be when PR goes to below 40, the period when the dollar was pegged to gold at $35 per ounce. With gold at $1000, silver could trade over $25 per ounce. It still would be trading at half the 1980 peak price of $50 per ounce. If gold goes to $2500 per ounce in about five years, as predicted by experts, silver could explode to over $70 per ounce. If PR goes below 20, as it had been when gold and silver were pegged to the currencies for over a hundred years before the twentieth century, the price of silver for every ounce could go over $100.

The second force that could propel the price upward is based upon the supply and demand fundamentals rather than currency changes or chart configurations. Alexander the Great is said to have used silver coins to purify water. The huge collection of impressionist art at the Barnes Foundation near Philadelphia had amassed a fortune built on selling an antiseptic silver compound called Argyrol in the early 20th century. Recently, **Pure Bioscience** (PURE), a El Cajon, California, company has a silver-based molecule it thinks can be used in a whole range of products, from cleaning products to agriculture to cosmetics and perhaps, someday as a drug. Silver has become a vital industrial metal, needed in thousands of industrial, high-tech, and medical applications, while gold remains true to its historical jewellery, investment and hedging roles.

This changing new dual-role for silver — both as a precious metal and an industrial necessity — resulted in a phenomenon unprecedented in the annals of history. This new demand for a universally known and revered commodity has almost evaporated the cumulative production of 5,000 years of world mining. Recall in India, silver coins, associated with Goddess Laxmi, are given as gifts on auspicious occasions. Who could have ever imagined that the silver being plundered and shipped from the Americas to Europe 400 years ago would be consumed in cellphones, TVs and water purifiers? Silver has become mandatory in all sorts of modern things designed to make life better. It has also created the investment opportunity of a lifetime, because there is unquestioned documentation, prepared by researchers like Theodore Butler, who has been monitoring silver market for decades, that not enough of this good news metal exists to go around.

Based upon the data given by United States Geological Survey (USGS, http://minerals.usgs.gov/minerals/pubs/commodity/), silver analyst Ted Butler claims that silver is the rarest of all important metals, including gold. This is based upon a unique geological circumstance, known as epithermal deposition, which holds that most of the silver in the earth's crust was deposited near the surface. As a result, there is less silver available the deeper we go. If he is correct, the price of silver should go exponentially high in years to come. That would mean that not only are we running out of above-ground silver, we are also running out of silver below ground much sooner than anyone has imagined. The statistics from the USGS are comprehensive and free of any known bias. All other available sources confirm the USGS data.

We know all mineral resources are finite in existence. While more resources may be discovered, no new mineral resources are actually being created. Once they are gone, they are gone for ever! We will always find and produce enough of everything, given the correct price encouragement. There is no way we can keep producing at current rates until the moment of complete depletion in any mineral. But the data indicates there are limits to what can be taken from the ground. And also the data clearly shows that there is less silver below ground relative to current production than any other metal. But the irony is that if the resource data are correct, higher production only reduces the number of years profitable silver will be available. Consequently, higher silver mine production would become extremely difficult.

There is another factor to be considered. If the world is running out of silver and other minerals due to depletion of below ground reserves then there will be changes in how the remaining reserves are valued and observed. Countries that are fortunate to hold the most of the surviving reserves will become more protective of those reserves and extract maximum value. This will increase the risk of taxation and nationalization to the mining companies. It will only improve the value of silver holdings.

In the current environment, commodities have underperformed in the last five months starting from the March 2009 market low. This is mainly due to the perception of deflation and the process of deleveraging through which we are going. However, the bankers of the world are pumping money into the system to insure that the world economy does not fall into the spiral of deflation that could result in depression. Sooner or later, they will succeed in bringing substantial inflation in the economy and that is when silver as an investment could do well.

The third force that could pressure on the silver price is government regulations. By the Commodity Exchange Act, position limits, which determine the amount of speculative trading allowed, exist to prevent unnecessary price fluctuation that could lead to later failures in contract settlement. For over a decade, silver's position limits greatly surpass those of other commodities. Even though the limit in COMEX silver is currently at 6,000 contracts, still exemptions are being made, causing severe manipulation of the silver market. The Commodity Futures Trading Commission (CFTC), a US Government agency, is not entirely responsible for this problem, though they are very likely involved. In the late 90s, the government curtailed its stringent directive in favour of the financial industry's own self-regulation. What seemed like a good idea resulted in excessive manipulation of the market by bullion banks. The bullion banks short both silver and gold far more than could actually be covered, very likely to control the perception of inflation. The logical cure for a potential tsunami in the future is to put CFTC back in charge of position limits, as no organisation would ever decide to limit its own power and profits. Now that we have experienced the bailouts galore and a huge stimulus package, CFTC is looking into putting back some reasonable control over gold and silver trading. This is to prevent bullion banks from getting into trouble, if the supply shortage of deliverable gold and silver develops.

In the modern age of instant communication, the whole world knows about the managed (manipulated) gold and silver market, and the out of control world reserve currency, the dollar. Countries like China are making legal and even encouraging the populace to hold gold and silver. Their leaders, claiming that we are now in a multi-polar world, want to replace the dollar with something else as the world reserve currency. It is apparent, at least in this writer's view, that silver has a great future.

August 2009

The Banyan Tree
Asia's Mascot

THE *Economist*'s first Asia-centered column titled "Banyan" was initiated on April 11th, 2009, comparable to columns "Lexington" for America and "Bagehot" for England. It continues the discourse about Asian issues, with an explanation of their concentration in spirituality and entrepreneurialism. Though the awareness that will be brought to readers is laudable, why is the spread of Asian values so important only now? Their answer is simple; this century is expected to be the Asian Century. The last intellectual push for pan-Asianism was promoted nearly a century ago by Rabindranath Tagore, a Nobel laureate. He was well received on tours to China and Japan, where he urged people to counter Western imperialism with an Asian spiritualism. However, he did not succeed then. There is no doubt about the perception among Western intellectuals like Carl Jung, among others, that spiritualism is strongly associated with the East, particularly with India. The international headquarters of the Theosophical Society (an organisation to unite world traditions) was transferred from New York to Adyar, Chennai, in the late 1870s because Adyar had one of the largest forests of banyan trees. Later, under the leadership of Annie Besant, they discovered in Adyar a Christ-like young boy named Krishnamurti, with, an aura of selflessness.

For centuries, Western countries have relied on and built upon the inventions and discoveries of the East. Some will argue that technology has been enhanced by innovation from Asia, such as rocketry. But this first article in "Banyan"; In the shade of the banyan tree" focuses on the romanticism of Western ideals by countries such as Japan, and says that the Asian spotlight on technology is more "imitation" than representation of "Asian identity". The article claims, and many of us will agree, that even more important are the spirituality and traditions of Asia, uncontaminated by the reliance on the West.

The article brings to attention the increase of Asia's exports within and to the West. This is a positive not only because of the growth of Asia's economic integration, but also because this supports the new concept that the "simultaneous rise of two continent-sized big powers can be peaceful." The magazine advocates friendly and constructive competition in place of destructive, as has occurred in the West. Very rarely do we consider multiple big powers a sign of anything but war and discontent, but it does not have to be so. For years the world has lived with its countries in discord and at each other's throats, for survival and affluence. How many years will it take to see that this way of dealing with other cultures and peoples hasn't been and is still not working? It is about time that we try something else. Every growing power has a breaking point, and until we find mediation, balance, harmony and complementarity, those powers will forever fail, as I have argued in my previous writings.

So why is the banyan tree the mascot for the Asian economy, culture and traditions? The tree is found both physically and spiritually in nearly all Asian countries. The tree is sacred in Hindu theology; for instance, we often see the God Shiva meditating under the shade of such a tree. It is often called "The Tree of Life" or "The Tree of Knowledge." It is simple to understand the former, its symbolism of eternal life, when considering the visual appearance of unending expansion. Vishnu is also said to have taught beneath a banyan trees, bringing knowledge of philosophy and science to the people. The Bodhi Tree, under which Buddha attained enlightenment, was a banyan by another name. A British magazine, by naming the column "Banyan", may be recognising that India is at the roots of all Asians, perhaps of all the world civilisations as many scholars of genetic research have hypothesised.

Not only is the banyan tree sprinkled throughout the various countries' mythology, religion and daily life, but the science of the tree itself is representative of the perpetual growth and vastness of Asia's branches. After the dispersal of the seeds from the banyan fruit, the roots erupt from the soil and spread laterally. Asia contains more than half the world's population, based upon the latest census. The people themselves span worldwide in respect to geographical location, political power, and cultural influence. Like the roots of the banyan, the massive Asian population grows strong and comes to resemble the core trunk from which they originated. The population, also like the roots, extends to all corners of the earth much farther than one initially imagines it could. The roots simultaneously lengthen and simultaneously cling to the host trunk and remain attached for all its life-span, continually adding to the trunk, the core, the ancient tradition, and creating new life elsewhere.

The picture associated with the article features a giant tree erupting from and spreading over a large portion of the earth. This tree's roots are not the only things to spread far over the land, for the branches are just as far-reaching. Even the parts of the world that are not home to the Asian people themselves are still "in the shade of the banyan tree," being affected by the continent and its inhabitants, however indirectly. The shade is immense, but through the leaves, here and there, the sky still shines through — its shade does not smother or trap one in darkness.

It is interesting to note that the name "Banyan" came from the writer's caste "Bania" derived from the Gujarati name "Va(ha)nias" meaning boat-businessmen travelling as far as Java and Sumatra. Among Gujaratis, baniya or vanias implies they are grocers or merchants by profession. The Portuguese picked up the word to refer specifically to Hindu merchants and passed it along to the English as early as 1599 with the same meaning. By 1634, English writers began to tell of the banyan tree, a tree under which Hindu merchants would conduct their business. The tree provided a shaded place for a village meeting or for merchants to sell their goods. Eventually, banyan came to mean the tree itself. Even today children are schooled under the banyan tree in some tribal areas. *The Times of India*, one of the largest newspapers in India, also has a column on spiritualism under the heading, "Under the Banyan Tree."

June 2009

Deepening Depression

As the currency carry trades swept away Iceland in 2007, and later bankers tried minimising the effect of sub-prime toxins in 2008, there is still no light at the end of the tunnel based upon the most recent data received in the first week of June 2009. The contradiction is that the stock market is singing a different, more optimistic tune. This might be because institutions like Goldman-Government Sachs (GGS) predict a brighter future by investing in the BRIC (Brazil, Russia, India, and China) countries and in energy. The word "Government" was introduced in the middle because they seem to be providing Treasury Secretaries and economic advisers to US Presidents for a couple of decades. GGS believes that the world economy will roar back on a tidal wave of liquidity and is forecasting that oil will rise to over $85 per barrel. Government seems to give an impression that the worst is behind us.

Contradicting that forecast, the executives of big oil companies state that the oil markets are awash with so much crude that about 100 million barrels are stored on tankers at sea. John Williams, who runs Shadow Government Statistics (www.shadowstats.com) thinks that we are experiencing Pollyanna Creep — Pollyanna being the orphan lead character of the 1913 children's book, who learns to find a cheery perspective on life's misery. Williams debunks government data and claims that the unemployment is over 20%, GDP is shrinking by 8% and CPI is up by 7%. He believes that the tidal wave of liquidity created by the government will result in a massive stagflation, much bigger than the one in 1970s. One does hear whispers from former government officers stating that there is always political pressure to manipulating data to their advantage.

Optimists think that the developing economies will pull us out of global recession. However, China, the main driver of the new economy, is using about 10% less electricity from a year earlier, in spite of the strong fiscal boost given by the Chinese government. Scholars of the depression era economy conclude that the global rupture over the last ten months has been more violent than during the earlier slumps because global debt leverage was much greater this time. The fall in world industrial output on average is worse compared to what happened during the 1929-1930 period of depression. The manufacturing capacity utilisation is running at a historic low of about 50 to 60%. The danger is that companies will have to fire a lot of workers, deepening deflation. Here in Los Angeles, corporations and institutions like UCLA are cutting costs and salaries of employees.

Stephen Roach of Morgan Stanley fears an Asian relapse because of Asia's fatal dependence on exports to the West. China's incipient economic rebound is based upon infrastructure spending. Apparently, that alone cannot be sufficient to pull the global economy out of the slump. The global economy that got used to American spending is getting very little help from Americans, as nearly 80 million baby boomers ferociously retrench their spending. Their saving rate has jumped from almost nothing to over 5% and may test 15%, the post-war peak. The Obama administration is hoping to bring back the old paradigm of Americans shopping till they drop. That may never come back as Americans are concerned about an uncertain future and their needs during retirement.

After 9/11, George Bush's first doctrine was based upon his statement, "either you are with us to fight terrorism, or you are against us supporting terrorism". This was one of the reasons to declare war on Saddam, a supporter of terror, and pre-emptive strike. His second doctrine was about spreading democracy. His words, "the survival of liberty in our land increasingly depends on the success of liberty in other lands," resonates with John Kennedy's words, "we shall pay any price, bear any burden, meet any hardship, and support any friend to assure the survival and success of liberty."

"It is difficult to deal with terrorism through non-violence," the Tibetan spiritual leader, the Dalai Lama, said delivering the Madhavrao Scindia Memorial Lecture in Delhi in January 2009. He termed terrorism as the worst kind of violence which is not carried by a few mad people but by those who are brilliant and educated. "They (terrorists) are brilliant and educated . . . but a strong ill-feeling is bred in them. Their minds are closed. Only way to tackle terrorism is through prevention." The head of the Tibetan government-in-exile left the audience stunned when he said "I love President George W Bush." He went on to add how he and the US President instantly struck a chord in their first meeting, most unlike politicians who take a while to develop close ties. "I told him 'I love you but some of your policies I oppose'."

The stock bull market of last three months has driven down the bond market with rising interest rates and the cost of energy. The bond revolt alone in the past has brought the economic recovery to a halt. Rising interest rates are bad for all businesses, particularly for the real estate market.

Standards for underwriting real estate loans have been tightened after going through the experience of the sub-prime loan fiasco. The five-year interest-only loans and balloon loans, which were originated over the 2004-07 periods will face strong barriers as they will be due for refinancing up to the end of 2012. The combination of required additional cash due to the lower market value and higher interest rates will lead to an increase in defaults. In this scenario the apartment market should be least affected, while the buildings used for retail should fare the worst, followed by hotel and office buildings. Rising unemployment takes a toll on consumer spending and the decline in the level of business and travel reduces hotel occupancies. The poor economic conditions, cost cutting, and lay-offs take a toll on office leases.

If the borrower has maintained the monthly payments and is able to continue to do so, banks may negotiate loan extensions in an effort to forestall foreclosures. Banks do not have an interest in repossessing properties and trying to sell in a depressed market. Currently, there is leverage all the way across the system and there is no way to extract capital from depressed value properties as it was possible in the previous cycle. The rise in defaults should continue unless by some miracle, the market finds a bottom and stabilises.

P.S.

Argument to keeping a stronger dollar by M. R. Venkatesh: (November 2008)

Obviously, what aids and sustains the US dollar is a "suspended sense of disbelief" amongst countries about the value of US dollar. Yet, common sense tells us that the excess supply will obviously result in a fall in the value of any product. The US dollar is no exception.

The late Iraqi leader Saddam Hussein was fully aware of this paradigm. Seeking to exploit the inherent weakness of the US dollar, Saddam wanted to trade his crude in euros, which would have lead to a lower demand for the US dollar and thereby triggered a dollar collapse. Those were his "weapons of mass destruction — WMD."

And if some analysts are to be believed, Venezuela and Iran too possess the very same WMDs. Naturally, it requires some specious arguments and/or military intervention to protect the US dollar. Never in the history of mankind has a national army protected the national currency so vigorously as the US Armilitary has done in the past decade or so.

June 2009

Inflation or Deflation?

As I have explained in my book, Saving Us From Ourselves, Nature always creates pairs of opposites everywhere, organisms and organisations included. As usual, there are two views among economists, while the government is trying hard at getting out of deflationary pressure by injecting trillions into the economic system. It is accurate to say that we have experienced deflation in the past several quarters. The state of the economy can be measured by four indicators constituting of two pairs of opposites tied to the four human attributes, as explained in my book. The four economic indicators are the rate of inflation (CPI), interest rates, GDP growth, and unemployment. We are experiencing deflation because the GDP growth is negative, CPI was about half a percent negative in the first quarter of this year, unemployment is approaching 10 per cent, and the treasury interest rate is being kept artificially close to zero. In essence, the wheels of the economy are slowing down, thanks to the imbalance in the pairs of economic indicators created by government manipulation.

Ben Bernanke, who did his PhD on the subject of the 1930s Depression, is known as "Helicopter Ben." He is known to have expressed his views that the way to resolve a depression is to print the money and throw it from a helicopter. The second group of economists believe that the Fed may not be able to control the rate of inflation, once the inflation rate starts climbing due to the trillions of dollars permeating the system. Inflation can be controlled by increasing interest rate as we saw in the 1980s. But they also believe that the Fed may not do so due to the political pressure and the fragile economy and the banking system.

So are we going to have Zimbabwe-style inflation or a Japanese-style deflation? In Zimbabwe, the lowest denominated paper note is cheaper than the toilet paper we use and the deflation in Japan has been lingering for the last two decades. Government and Wall Street are trying hard to convey the perception that the worst is behind us. After all, the psychology is the most important factor in navigating markets.

In time, Bernanke should have his way and we should be out of deflation and enter the domain of inflation; no one knows how long it will take, though. However, we need to accept the fact that the old glory days are gone for good as far in the future as we can see. Why? The process of deleveraging has impaired consumers and financial institutions. The trend of the last 25 years of "borrow and spend" has been replaced by the old ways of "saving for a rainy day". The financial system is damaged severely due to the vaporisation of virtual banks like hedge funds and insurance companies holding worthless toxic assets. The growth in the domestic demand in Western countries will not be as good as in emerging markets. Emerging markets crashed along with the Western markets because their exports to the West had dwindled. However, they have a great potential in enlarging their middle class.

The trend towards worrisome inflation is here to stay. Nations around the globe have adopted the Keynesian currency printing experiment; we have never seen such unanimity among nations ever in history in going for Keynesian economic philosophy. There are reputable economists who believe that we cannot get out of deflation for years to come. There is another trend developing; for example, China has converted their dollars into commodities like copper, silver and gold; essentially, commodities becoming a parallel world reserve currency. Commodities could become a dominant currency only if inflation takes off.

The current economic quagmire, the people at GATA (Gold Anti-Trust Action Committee) believe, is due to the manipulation of gold and silver prices by bullion banks with the blessings of the Fed and the government. Bullion banks buy, or lease gold from various sources and sell to generate profit. GATA, in essence, is the opposite of the Fed in a nature's pair and is an education and civil rights organisation with a goal to force governments to implement free market for all goods and services, including gold and silver. They also believe that loose money policy always creates market bubbles in due course. Gold price, if traded freely, becomes an alarm signal on the world economy system; it indicates the "nutritional value" of the currency, literally. Gold, in essence, acts as a reference or an anchor to bring balance and stability to the movement of the currency. In the 1970s when it was freely traded, it gave a strong signal of inflation. Fed chairman Paul Volcker was able to bring inflation down, strengthening the dollar. Had the gold price not been suppressed by bullion banks in the last two decades, they would have given a strong signal long before the credit bubbles brought the world economy crashing down. The Achilles' Heel of the bullion banks is the shortage of physical gold and silver.

There are only two possible outcomes as I see it. Either the bullion banks will fail in the end, or the US government will have destroyed what remains of the free market in America. I hope it is the former, but the continuing flow of events from Washington, D.C. and the actions of policymakers suggest it could be the latter.

May 2009

Bibliography

Baker, W. Raymond, *Capitalism's Achilles Heel*, New Jersey: John Wiley & Sons, Inc., 2005

Batra, Ravi, *The New Golden Age*, New York: Palgrave Macmillan, 2007.

Batra, Ravi, *Greenspan's Fraud*, New York: Palgrave Macmillan, 2005.

Batra, Ravi, *Common Sense Macroeconomics*, Dallas: Liberty Press, 2005.

Batra, Ravi, *The Crash of the Millennium*, New York: Random House, 1999.

Batra, Ravi, *The Great American Deception*, New York: John Wiley & Sons, 1996.

Berstein, Peter, I., *Capital Ideas*, New York: The Free Press, a division of Macmillan, 1992.

Black, John, *Oxford Dictionary of Economics*, Oxford and New York: Oxford University Press, 1997, 2002.

Das, Satyajit, *Traders Guns & Money*, England: Perason, 2010.

Davies, Glyn, *A History of Money: From Ancient Times to the Present Day*, Cardiff: University of Wales Press, 1994.

Doshi, Navin, *Transcedence: Saving Us from Ourselves*, New York: Ithaca Press, 2009.

Greenspan, Alan, *The Age of Turbulence*, New York: The Penguin Press, 2007.

Hayek, F.A., *The Road to Serfdom*, London: The University of Chicago Press, 2007.

Heilbroner, L. Robert and Lester C. Thurow, *Economics Explained*, New York: Simon & Schuster, Inc., 1987.

Jastram, W. Roy, *The Golden Constant*, New York: Ronald Press Publication: John Wiley & Sons Inc., 1977.

Jung, C.G., *A Physical Approach to the Dogma of the Trinity*, 1942 in Collected Works, Vol. II.

Kanth, Rajani, *The Challenge of Eurocentrism: Global Perspectives, Policy, and Prospects*, New York: Macmillan, 2009.

Kaufman, Henry, *Interest Rates, the Markets, and the New Financial World*, New York: Times Books, a division of Random House Inc., 1986.

Koch, Richard, *The 80/20 Principle*, New York: Doubleday, 1998.

Kuhn, Thomas, *The Structure of Scientific Revolution*, Chicago: University of Chicago Press, 1996.

Kumar, Nirmal, *The Tao of Psychology*, Bombay: Bharatiya Vidhya Bhavan, 1993.

Mandlebrot, Benoit, and Richard Hudson, *The (Mis) Behavior of Markets*, New York: Basic Books, 2004.

Pearce, W. David, *The MTT Dictionary of Modern Economics*, Massachusetts, The MIT Press, 1992.

Rajan, G. Raghuram, *Fault Lines*, Princeton & Oxford: Princeton University Press, 2010.

Rajan, G. Raghuram & Luigi Zingales, *Saving Capitalism from the Capitalists*, New York: Crown Business, 2003.

Rangarajan, L.N., *Kautliya: The Arthashastra*, New Delhi: Penguin Books, 1987.

Rucker, Rudy, *Mind Tools*, Boston, Houghton Miffin Company, 1987.

Sowell, Thomas, *Basic Economics*, New York: Basic Books, 2000.

Taleb, Nicholas Nassim, *The Black Swan: The Impact of the Highly Improbable*, New York: Random House, 2007.

Index